Intraocular Lens

*Edited by Xiaogang Wang
and Felicia M. Ferreri*

Published in London, United Kingdom

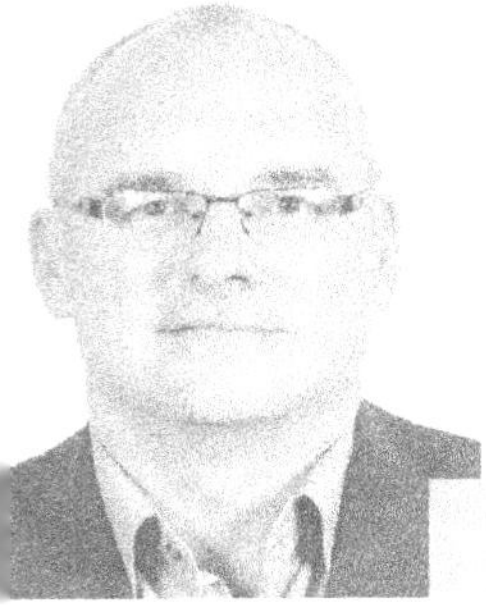

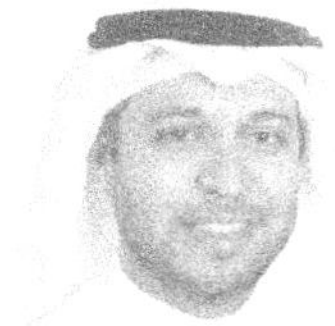

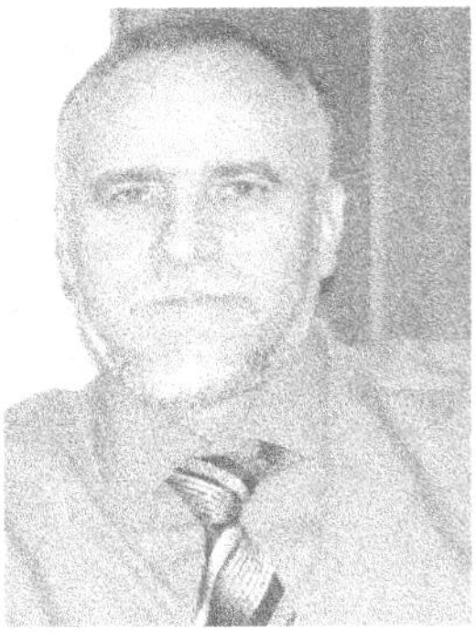

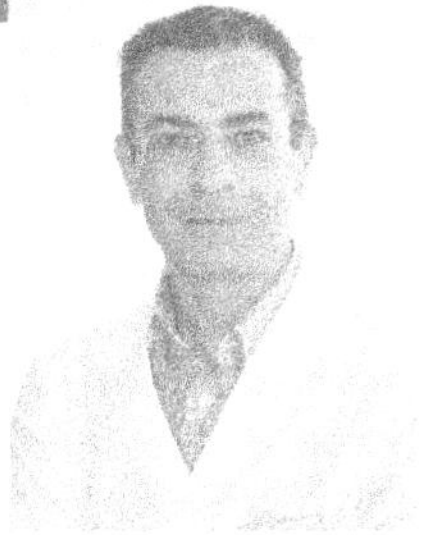

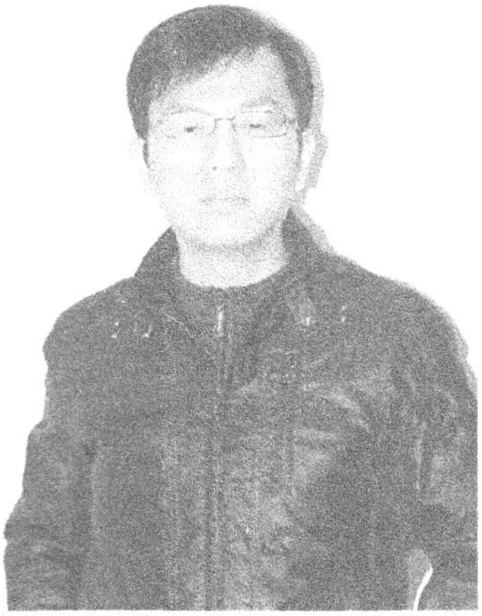

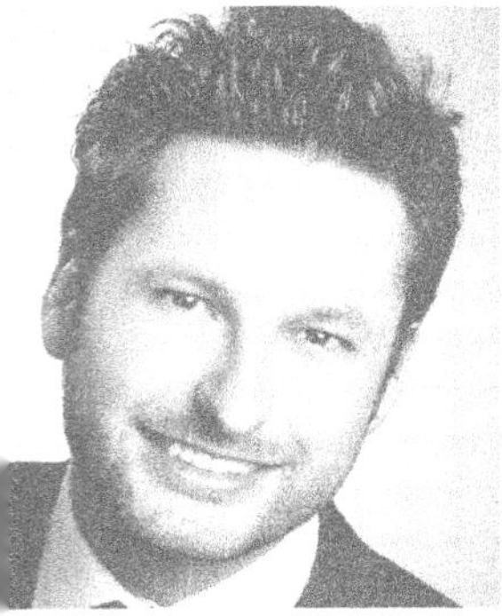

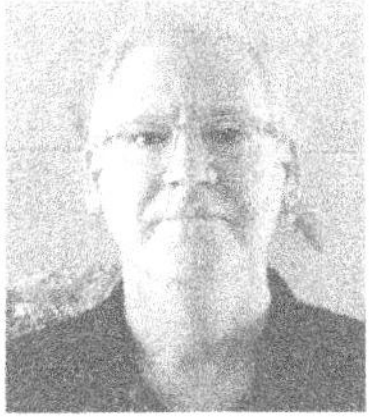

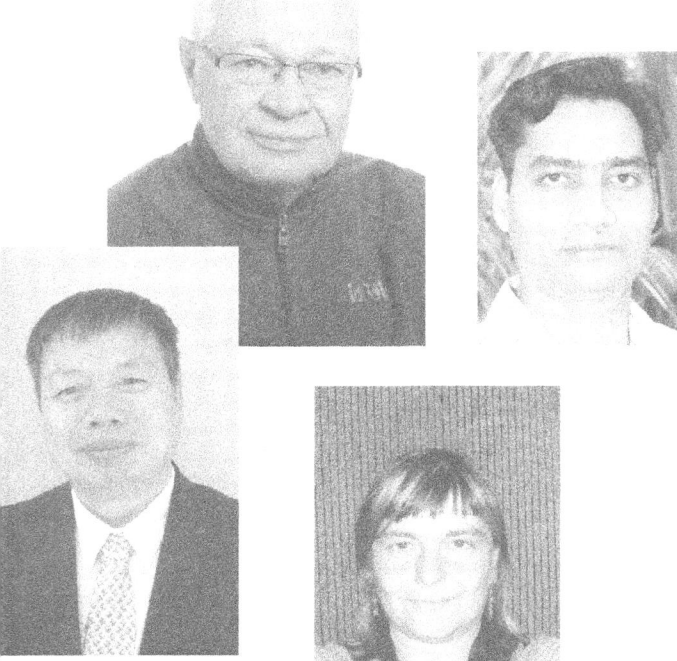
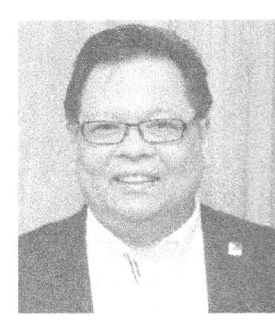
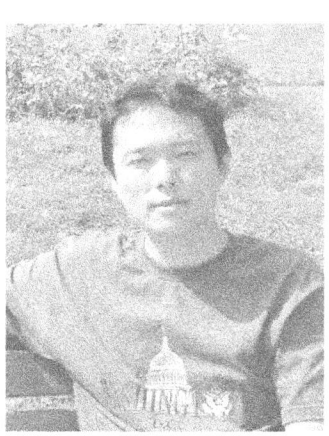

IntechOpen

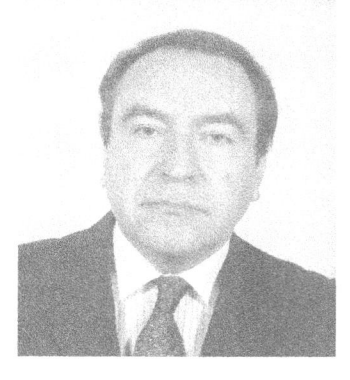
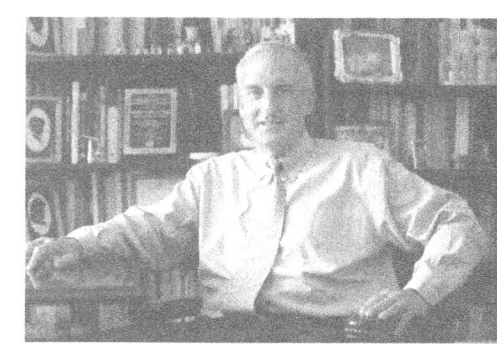
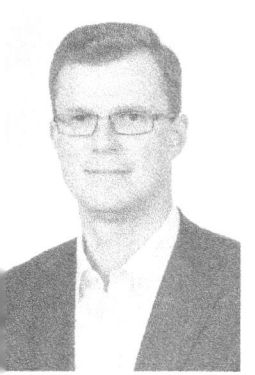
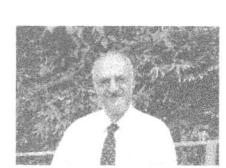
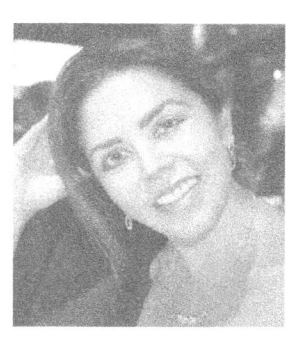

Supporting open minds since 2005

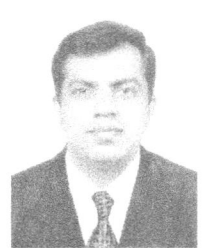
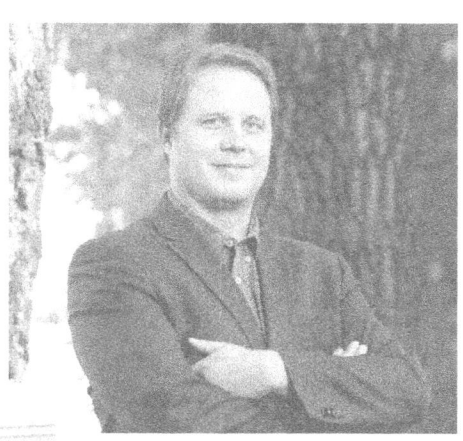
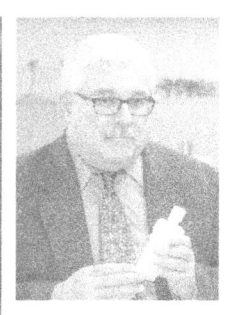
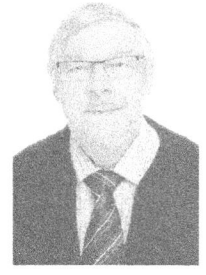
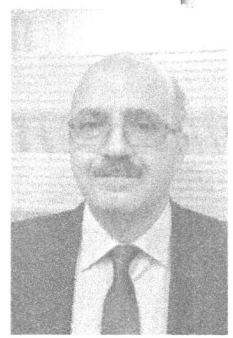
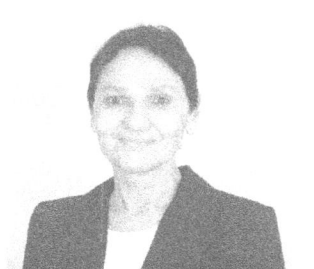
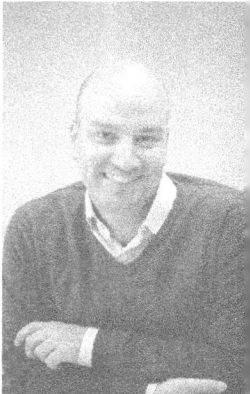

Intraocular Lens
http://dx.doi.org/10.5772/intechopen.79001
Edited by Xiaogang Wang and Felicia M. Ferreri

Contributors
Enzo Maria Vingolo, Giuseppe Napolitano, Lorenzo Casillo, Maja Bohac, Maja Pauk-Gulic, Alma Biscevic, Ivan Gabric, Sangeethabalasri Pugazhendhi, Allan Hunter, Balamurali Ambati, Timo Eppig, Achim Langenbucher, Jens Schrecker, Arthur Messner, Emely Zoraida Karam Aguilar, Zequan Xu, Suzana Konjevoda, Samir Čanović, Ana Didović Pavičić, Robert Stanić, Simona-Delia Delia Nicoara, Pradeep Prasad, Niranjan Manoharan, Smita Kapoor, Shreya Gupta

© The Editor(s) and the Author(s) 2020
The rights of the editor(s) and the author(s) have been asserted in accordance with the Copyright, Designs and Patents Act 1988. All rights to the book as a whole are reserved by INTECHOPEN LIMITED. The book as a whole (compilation) cannot be reproduced, distributed or used for commercial or non-commercial purposes without INTECHOPEN LIMITED's written permission. Enquiries concerning the use of the book should be directed to INTECHOPEN LIMITED rights and permissions department (permissions@intechopen.com).
Violations are liable to prosecution under the governing Copyright Law.

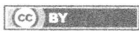

Individual chapters of this publication are distributed under the terms of the Creative Commons Attribution 3.0 Unported License which permits commercial use, distribution and reproduction of the individual chapters, provided the original author(s) and source publication are appropriately acknowledged. If so indicated, certain images may not be included under the Creative Commons license. In such cases users will need to obtain permission from the license holder to reproduce the material. More details and guidelines concerning content reuse and adaptation can be found at http://www.intechopen.com/copyright-policy.html.

Notice
Statements and opinions expressed in the chapters are these of the individual contributors and not necessarily those of the editors or publisher. No responsibility is accepted for the accuracy of information contained in the published chapters. The publisher assumes no responsibility for any damage or injury to persons or property arising out of the use of any materials, instructions, methods or ideas contained in the book.

First published in London, United Kingdom, 2020 by IntechOpen
IntechOpen is the global imprint of INTECHOPEN LIMITED, registered in England and Wales, registration number: 11086078, 7th floor, 10 Lower Thames Street, London,
EC3R 6AF, United Kingdom
Printed in Croatia

British Library Cataloguing-in-Publication Data
A catalogue record for this book is available from the British Library

Additional hard and PDF copies can be obtained from orders@intechopen.com

Intraocular Lens
Edited by Xiaogang Wang and Felicia M. Ferreri
p. cm.
Print ISBN 978-1-83880-484-8
Online ISBN 978-1-83880-485-5
eBook (PDF) ISBN 978-1-78923-830-3

We are IntechOpen,
the world's leading publisher of Open Access books
Built by scientists, for scientists

4,900+
Open access books available

123,000+
International authors and editors

140M+
Downloads

151
Countries delivered to

Our authors are among the
Top 1%
most cited scientists

12.2%
Contributors from top 500 universities

WEB OF SCIENCE™

Selection of our books indexed in the Book Citation Index
in Web of Science™ Core Collection (BKCI)

Interested in publishing with us?
Contact book.department@intechopen.com

Numbers displayed above are based on latest data collected.
For more information visit www.intechopen.com

Meet the editors

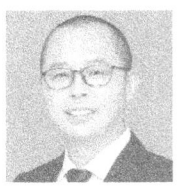

Dr. Xiaogang Wang joined the Shanxi Medical University Shanxi Eye Hospital in 2014 and was awarded the master postgraduate tutor of Shanxi Medical University in 2019. Dr. Wang earned his MD degree from Shanxi Medical University and a PhD degree from Shanghai Jiao Tong University. Dr. Wang completed his international fellowship on optical coherence tomography angiography with Dr. David Huang at the Casey Eye Institute in 2013. Dr. Wang was awarded 2 National Natural Science Foundation of China research project grants that support works that demonstrated clinical application of OCT/OCTA in cataract and artificial intelligence in IOL power calculation. He has published 30 peer-reviewed journal articles and 3 book chapters on ophthalmology.

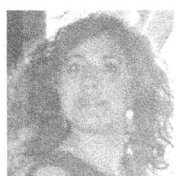

Felicia M. Ferreri graduated summa cum laude from the University of Messina, Italy in 1998 and completed her ophthalmology residency at the Policlinico Universitario, Messina in 2002. She was interned at San Raffaele Hospital in Milan (Corneal Section) and at the Hospital Careggi in Florence (pediatric ophthalmology diseases). She spent research periods in Seville (Virginio del Rocio Hospital), Madrid (San Carlos Hospital), Manchester (The Bolton Hospital), and Rio de Janiero (Universidade Fluminense). She has served as co-investigator for many national and international clinical trials. Since 2002, she has been Assistant Professor in Ophthalmology at the University of Messina. Her research interests are in the areas of glaucoma, neuro-ophthalmology, pediatric ophthalmology, and cataracts. She has authored more than 50 scientific papers.

Contents

Preface — XI

Section 1
Intraocular Lens Materials and Design — 1

Chapter 1
Basic Science of Intraocular Lens Materials — 3
by Smita Kapoor and Shreya Gupta

Chapter 2
Intraocular Lens (IOL) Materials — 13
by Samir Čanović, Suzana Konjevoda, Ana Didović Pavičić and Robert Stanić

Section 2
Aberration and Astigmatism Correction with Intraocular Lens — 21

Chapter 3
Aberration Correction with Aspheric Intraocular Lenses — 23
by Timo Eppig, Jens Schrecker, Arthur Messner and Achim Langenbucher

Chapter 4
Toric Intraocular Lenses — 35
by Zequan Xu

Section 3
Entoptic Phenomenon of Intraocular Lens — 51

Chapter 5
Pseudophakic Dysphotopsia — 53
by Emely Zoraida Karam Aguilar

Section 4
Myopia and Phakic Intraocular Lens — 65

Chapter 6
Pathologic Myopia: Complications and Visual Rehabilitation — 67
by Enzo Maria Vingolo, Giuseppe Napolitano and Lorenzo Casillo

Chapter 7 89
Reduction of Myopia Burden and Progression
by Sangeethabalasri Pugazhendhi, Balamurali Ambati and Allan A. Hunter

Chapter 8 101
Surgical Correction of Myopia
by Maja Bohac, Maja Pauk Gulic, Alma Biscevic and Ivan Gabric

Section 5
Secondary Intraocular Lens Techniques 121

Chapter 9 123
Secondary Intraocular Lens
by Niranjan Manoharan and Pradeep Prasad

Chapter 10 135
Scleral-Fixated Intraocular Lens: Indications and Results
by Simona-Delia Nicoară

Preface

Cataract surgery is one of the most frequently performed surgical procedures in the world. Intraocular lens (IOL), as an integral part of ocular refractive system reconstruction, is playing a more and more important role in cataract surgery. Moreover, with the development of IOL technology and patients' increasing demands of postoperative visual quality, different kinds of premium IOLs, such as the toric IOL, multifocal IOL, trifocal IOL, accommodating IOL, and extended depth of focus IOL, are widely used in ophthalmology. The careful and exact understanding of the optical physical properties of each type of IOL, their advantages and disadvantages, and biocompatibilities is essential.

This book is fortunate to have outstanding contributors from different countries. We believe that IOL content has a practical and clinical interest for clinical ophthalmology. Moreover, we hope that this book provides a timely answer to a current clinical need.

Xiaogang Wang, MD, PhD
Department of Ophthalmology,
Shanxi Eye Hospital,
Taiyuan, China

Felicia M. Ferreri, MD
Department BIOMORF,
University of Messina,
Messina, Italy

Section 1
Intraocular Lens Materials and Design

Chapter 1

Basic Science of Intraocular Lens Materials

Smita Kapoor and Shreya Gupta

Abstract

This chapter will explain the materials used in making intraocular lenses. Rigid IOL's made of PMMA have now given way to foldable silicone and acrylic lenses. This chapter will also throw light on the indications and contraindications for using each of the IOL's. The composition of each of the lenses, their water content, mechanical properties and their special ultraviolet absorbing features will be discussed in detail. The mechanism by which hydrophilic lenses are inserted through small incisions during cataract surgery will need a special mention. The problems with use of different types of intraocular lenses will also be dealt with.

Keywords: intraocular lens, material, PMMA, acrylic, silicone

1. Introduction

Cataract surgery is being carried out for over more than 3000 years. What began as simply dislodging the cataractous lens posteriorly into the vitreous, also known as couching, got the ball rolling. And now we have advanced surgical techniques with minimal incision size and excellent visual prognosis due to the recent advances in intraocular lenses (IOL) [1].

In November, 1949, Dr. Harold Ridley implanted the first intraocular lens after extracapsular cataract extraction (ECCE) in a 45 year old female at St. Thomas Hospital, London [2]. This IOL was made of a material called Polymethylmethacrylate (PMMA).

After a lot of clinical trials and initial disapproval, it wasn't until 1970, that IOL implantation became a well accepted procedure. And hence began a revolution in the field of cataract management. Over the past 5 decades there have been monumental breakthroughs and various IOLs of finest elements are now routinely being implanted (**Figure 1**).

An intraocular lens can be described on the basis of certain properties possessed by the material it is made up of. These properties include the following:

1. Affinity for water

2. Refractive index

3. Size of optic and haptic

4. Adhesiveness

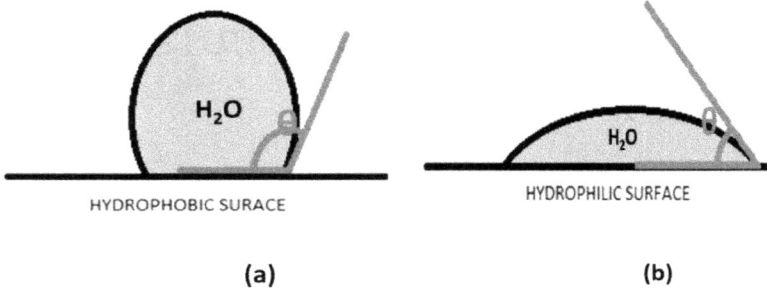

Figure 1.
Contact angles of water on hydrophobic and hydrophilic surfaces. (a) Contact angle is >90° on hydrophobic surface (b) contact angle is <90° on hydrophilic surface.

5. Presence or absence of glistening phenomenon

6. Prevention of posterior capsular opacification (PCO)

7. IOL design

1.1 Affinity for water

IOL materials are defined hydrophobic or hydrophilic according to the angle a drop of water makes with respect to the material surface. The more acute this angle is, the more hydrophilic the material is defined and vice versa.

1.2 Refractive index

Refractive index of a material refers to ratio of velocity of light in vacuum to velocity of light in that medium. It is a measure of bending of light rays when they travel through a particular medium. The refractive index and thickness of the IOL are inversely proportional.

1.3 Size

The optic diameter and the length of the haptics are taken into consideration when the size of the IOL is to be measured. The size of the incision, the type of injector and methods of introducing the IOL are all based on the size of the IOL.

1.4 Adhesiveness

Adhesiveness is a property by which the IOL fuses with anterior and posterior capsule and hence reduces the risk of decentration. This property becomes essential in toric IOLs.

1.5 Glistening phenomenon

Penetration by aqueous humor has been noted to cause small vacuoles within the lens optic. This phenomenon is called 'glistening phenomenon'.

1.6 Prevention of PCO

The properties of the IOL such as affinity for water, adhesiveness and presence of square edge contribute in prevention of opacification of posterior capsule after cataract surgery.

1.7 IOL design

The structure and design of IOL contributes to its ability to remain centered in the capsular bag. The shape and length of haptics and the optical diameter are taken into consideration in designing an intraocular lens.

2. Classification

Based on the materials, intraocular lenses can be classified as:

1. Rigid (PMMA)

2. Flexible (Silicone)

3. Foldable (Acrylic)

4. Collamer

2.1 PMMA

One of the first materials to be used for the purpose of intraocular lenses, polymethyl methacrylate (PMMA) is a rigid, non-foldable, hydrophobic material (**Figure 2**). Hydrophobic nature of PMMA lenses makes them more likely to adhere to corneal endothelial cells during insertion, thus causing potential endothelial loss. The refractive index is 1.49 and the usual optic diameter is 5–7 mm. They are usually single piece and have low memory haptics.

Due to their property of rigidity, a large incision is required for its implantation. An incision size of about 5.5–6 mm or a large corneoscleral tunnel is required for its

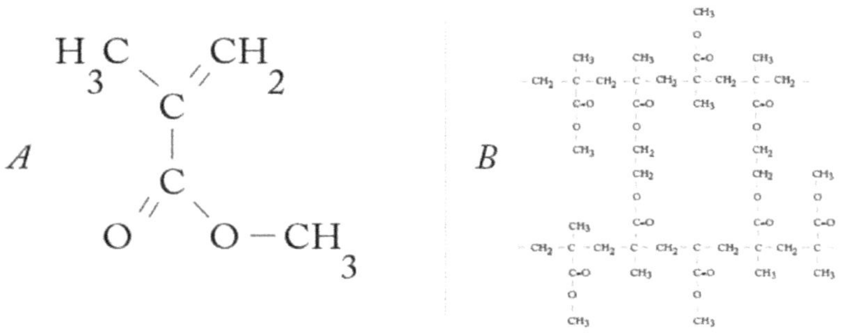

Figure 2.
(a) MMA (methyl methacrylate) forms the basis for acrylic IOLs. (b) Poly(methyl methacrylate) (PMMA) is a transparent thermoplastic; it was initially developed as a lightweight and shatter-resistant alternative to glass.

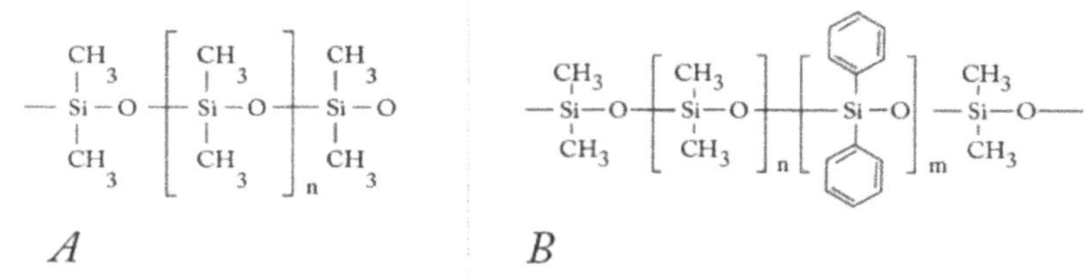

Figure 3.
(a) Polydimethylsiloxane and (b) polydimethyldiphenylsiloxane.

implantation. Large sized incisions are associated with delayed healing and astigmatic refractive errors. Hence PMMA is seldom used today except in developing countries due to economic reasons.

One piece variant of PMMA lens means that optics and haptics are made from a single mold of the same material. It is said to be three piece when the optics and the haptics are made from different materials and are attached together (**Figure 3**).

Penetration by aqueous humor has been noted to cause small vacuoles within the lens optic. This "glistening" phenomenon is rarely seen with PMMA.

After the advent of phacoemulsification in 1967, by Charles Kelman, the size of the incision did decrease significantly. However, the incision still had to be extended for implantation of the rigid IOL. The obligation of downsized incision was still amateur. This made way for the flexible and foldable breed of IOLs.

2.2 Silicone

Since 1950s, silicone has been used in a variety of medical device applications including contact and intraocular lenses. The malleable nature of silicone makes it chemically stable as well as imparts diverse mechanical properties. Also, due to its excellent biocompatibility and versatile properties, desired optical clarity and specific viscosity can be attained.

The first foldable silicone IOL was implanted in human eyes in the 1978 by Kai-yi Zhou. Silicone is hydrophobic, that is, it makes a contact angle of 99^0 with the water droplet on its material surface and therefore must be handled dry before implantation. This property allows a smaller incision than the IOL size. The refractive index of silicone lens is between 1.41 and 1.46 and the optic diameter is 5.5–6.5 mm. Because of the low refractive index, the optics are rather thick especially for high refractive powers. Such lenses may require an incision of size up to 3.2 mm. Although there are injectors available for safe and dry handling of silicone lenses, premature and abrupt opening of the lenses remains a dispute for most surgeons.

After implantation, the anterior capsule rim opacifies quickly, while the posterior capsule may remain clear for many years. Despite the low posterior capsular opacification (PCO) rate and the good resistance to Nd:YAG laser shots, silicone is less used today because it is not suitable for micro incision cataract surgery (MICS).

Adhesiveness is a property by which the IOL fuses with anterior and posterior capsule and hence reduces the risk of decentration. An important point about silicone lenses is that it has poor adhesive property and it is kept in place by the virtue of its haptics and capsule coalescence. The character of "glistening" is seen in silicone lenses as well.

Silicone lenses are available in two variants depending on the type of haptics. The two kinds of haptics include modified C loop and plate haptics. Of these, the plate haptics have a higher tendency to decenter in eyes with defective anterior capsule [3].

Silicone is a synthetic polymer made up of periodically repeated silicon-oxygen-groups (siloxane). This structure is the backbone for a polymer, which is identical for all silicone IOLs. Bound to the silicon atom are side chains, which influence the properties of the material.

2.3 Acrylic

The rigid PMMA lens is acrylic in nature. However the side chain molecules attached to the main polymer confer certain properties to the IOL. So, substituting the side chains in PMMA to hydroxyethyl or polyethyl groups alters the rigidity of the material. The newly formed polymers are now flexible and clear and this is the material that makes newer generation IOLs foldable. Furthermore, depending on the side-chain chemistry, the flexible acrylic material can be made to be hydrophilic or hydrophobic.

Most hydrophilic IOLs utilize the same material as contact lenses: hydroxyethylmethacrylate (HEMA) (**Figure 4**). Poly HEMA containing IOLs are also called hydrogels. With a water content of approximately 38%, they are flexible. Because of the high water content, they have a low refractive index. These lenses are highly foldable and can be injected through incisions approximately 1.8 mm in length or smaller, allowing for microincision cataract surgery (MICS). Because of hydrophilic nature of hydrogels, they are flexible and inert. Hydrophobic lenses have a low water content (<1%) and they carry a lesser risk of posterior capsule opacification. Higher uveal biocompatibility was achieved with the modern hydrophilic acrylic IOLs than with the hydrophobic acrylic IOL [4].

A salient property of these acrylic materials is glass transition temperature or Tg. It is essentially the temperature at which the material changes its rigidity and becomes more flexible. Tg is different for different acrylic materials depending on its side chain molecule.

Foldable acrylic lenses tend to be more robust than their silicone equivalents. They undergo less post-implantation decentration or rotation. If posterior segment surgery is likely to be necessary at a later date, they are a better choice, as silicone oil – which would ruin silicone-based IOLs – can be used. However, this comes at the cost of a slightly larger incision size being necessary for implantation.

The three piece hydrophobic acrylic foldable intraocular lens consists of a truncated hydrophobic optic and polymethylmethacrylate (PMMA) haptics. The single piece IOL is a new version of the hydrophobic acrylic foldable IOL, with both

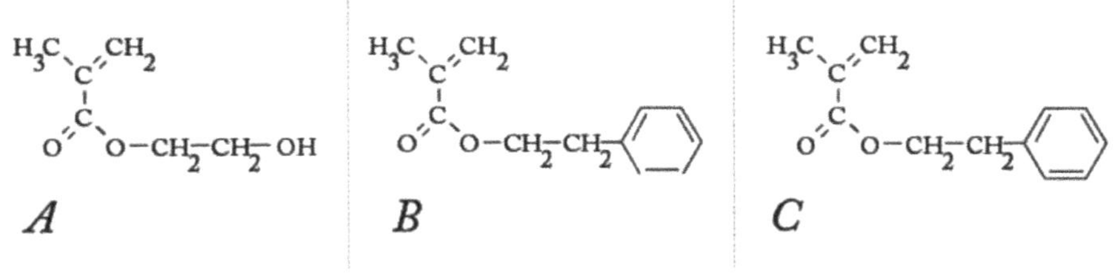

Figure 4.
Flexible acrylic lenses can be made from (a) HEMA – (hydroxyethyl) methacrylate, (b) PEMA – (polyethyl) methacrylate, and (c) PEA – poly(ethyl acrylate).

the optic and haptics consisting of a foldable acrylic material. The table below gives a comparison based on their different properties [5, 6]:

IOL Material	Advantage	Disadvantage
Hydrophilic acrylic	Higher tissue compatibility due to high water content Low aqueous flare Low rate of inflammatory cell accumulation on the lens surface	Insufficient posterior sharp-edged design due to the high water content High rate of posterior capsule opacification High rate of anterior capsule opacification Greater lens epithelial cell ongrowth on the lens surface
Hydrophobic acrylic	Material compatible with a posterior sharp-edged design Low rate of posterior capsule opacification Low rate of anterior capsule opacification Low rate of lens epithelial cell ongrowth on the lens surface	High aqueous flare* Inflammatory cell accumulation on the lens surface*
PMMA	Good tissue compatibility Low aqueous flare Low rate of inflammatory cell accumulation on the lens surface	Foldable High rate of posterior capsule opacification
Silicone	Low rate of inflammatory cell accumulation on the lens surface Low rate of posterior capsule opacification	Increased fibrotic reaction due to lens epithelial cell stimulation Lens surface opacification due to contact with intravitreal air Difficulty visualizing the retina due to interface formed with silicone oil used in vitreoretinal surgery

*Not at a clinically significant level
PMMA: Poly(methylmethacrylate); IOL: Intraocular lenses

Properties	Single piece acrylic	Three piece acrylic
Visual acuity	Same	Same
Refractive stability	Same	Same
Centration	Same	Same
SPCO formation	More	Less
Anterior capsule opacification	Less	More
Dysphotopsias	Less	More

	PMMA	Silicone	Acrylic
Size	5–7 mm	5.5–6.5 mm	Foldable (minimum 1.8 mm)
Rigidity	Rigid	Flexible	Foldable
Affinity to water	hydrophobic	hydrophobic	Hydrophilic/hydrophobic
Refractive index	1.49	1.41–1.46	1.39–1.42

2.4 Collamer

Another subset of hydrophilic foldable acrylics is the Collamer lens. This Collamer material is a patented copolymer of hydrophilic acrylic and porcine collagen (<0.1%) hydroxyethyl methacrylate copolymer with a UV absorbing chromophore. In theory, the porcine collagen improves the biocompatibility of the lens when implanted in human eyes. It is a foldable phakic IOL consisting of a plate haptic with a central convex/concave optical zone and a forward vault to reduce the contact with the lens.

3. Ultraviolet absorbing intraocular lenses

The crystalline lens absorbs ultraviolet radiation between 300 and 400 nm and protects the retina from photochemical damage [7]. This protective phenomenon is lost when the lens is removed during cataract surgery, but it can be restored by the implanting a UV-absorbing polymethylmethacrylate IOL. Implantation of a UV absorbing IOL results in cyanopsia or blue tinted vision. However it helps in preventing age related macular degeneration, improving contrast sensitivity and

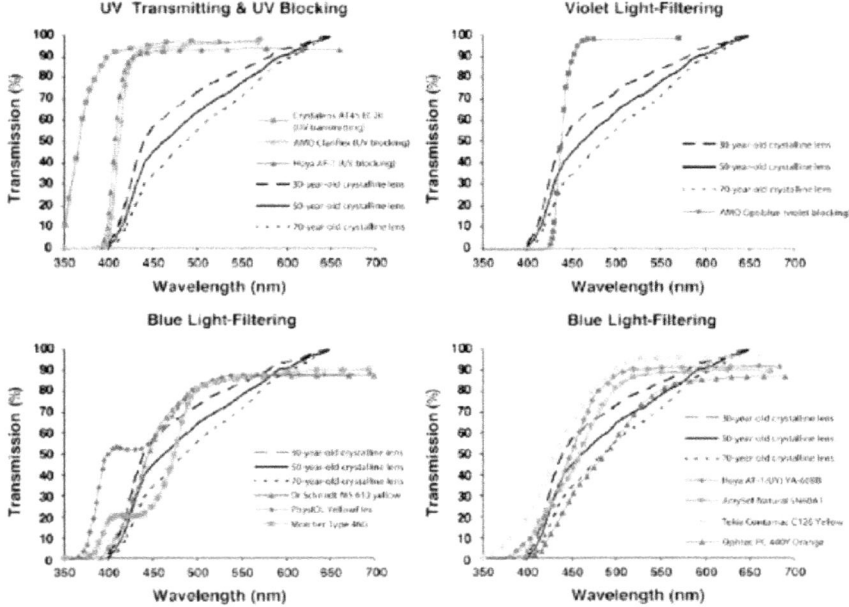

Figure 5.
Comparison of transmission spectra of UV transmitting, UV blocking, violet light-filtering and blue light-filtering IOLs [8, 9].

reducing glare in mesopic and photopic conditions. There are various UV-absorbing IOLs but they are not equally effective in absorbing UV radiation (**Figure 5**). To prevent the toxic effects of short wavelength light, IOL's have been developed that only block UV light but also reduce transmission of violet and blue wavelengths. The yellow pigment containing IOL's were first developed by Hoya in Japan followed by Menicon Co. Ltd. The first foldable IOL was developed by Alcon Laboratories.

4. Future aspects

The incidence of endophthalmitis following cataract surgery has reduced significantly over the last few decades but it is still a nightmare for every eye surgeon. Post-operative instillation of topical antibiotics and antiinflammatory is the rule. However, recent studies show that delivery of these drugs intraocularly released from the IOL material may reduce the need for postoperative medication and thereby may further reduce the incidence of endophthalmitis. A combination of moxifloxacin and ketorolac is better than a combination of moxifloxacin with diclofenac [10]. Its effective against *Staph. aureus* and *Staph. epidermidis* for about 15 days. Further studies should be aimed at such modern dual drug delivery incorporated in the IOL.

5. Summary

Right from couching and rendering the patient aphakic, science has come a long way to manufacturing intraocular lens. The different materials have their own advantages and pitfalls owing to their chemical structure and inherent properties. UV absorbing and dual drug delivery systems are the future.

Author details

Smita Kapoor* and Shreya Gupta
Vision Eye Centre, New Delhi, India

*Address all correspondence to: smitakapoor21@yahoo.in

IntechOpen

© 2020 The Author(s). Licensee IntechOpen. This chapter is distributed under the terms of the Creative Commons Attribution License (http://creativecommons.org/licenses/by/3.0), which permits unrestricted use, distribution, and reproduction in any medium, provided the original work is properly cited.

References

[1] Kumari R, Srivastava M, Garg P, Janardhanan R. Intra ocular lens technology – A review of journey from its inception. Ophthalmology Research: An International Journal. 2020:1-9. DOI: 10.9734/or/2019/v11i330129

[2] Davis G. The evolution of cataract surgery. Missouri Medicine. 2016;**113**(1):58-62

[3] Zhou KY. Silicon intraocular lenses in 50 cataract cases. Chinese Medical Journal. 1983;**96**(3):175-176

[4] Özyol P, Özyol E, Karel F. Biocompatibility of intraocular lenses. Turkish Journal of Ophthalmology. 2017;**47**(4):221-225. DOI: 10.4274/tjo.10437

[5] Nejima R, Miyata K, Honbou M, et al. A prospective, randomised comparison of single and three piece acrylic foldable intraocular lenses. The British Journal of Ophthalmology. 2004;**88**(6):746-749. DOI: 10.1136/bjo.2003.037663

[6] Chang DF. Single versus three piece acrylic IOLs. The British Journal of Ophthalmology. 2004;**88**(6):727-728. DOI: 10.1136/bjo.2004.040063

[7] Sparrow JR, Miller AS, Zhou J. Blue light-absorbing intraocular lens and retinal pigment epithelium protection in vitro. Journal of Cataract and Refractive Surgery. 2004;**30**:873-878

[8] Fiona C, Stuart P, Katharina W, Russell F, Susan D. Blue light-filtering intraocular lenses: Review of potential benefits and side effects. Journal of Cataract and Refractive Surgery. 2009;**35**:1281-1297. DOI: 10.1016/j.jcrs.2009.04.017

[9] Nilsson SEG, Textorius O, Andersson B-E, Swenson B. Clear PMMA versus yellow intraocular lens material. An electrophysiologic study on pigmented rabbits regarding "the blue light hazard". Progress in Clinical and Biological Research. 1989;**314**:539-553

[10] Ana T, Serro AP, Saramago B. Dual drug delivery from intraocular lens material for prophylaxis of endophthalmitis in cataract surgery. International Journal of Pharmaceutics. 2019;**558**:43-52. DOI: 10.1016/j.ijpharm.2018.12.028

Chapter 2

Intraocular Lens (IOL) Materials

Samir Čanović, Suzana Konjevoda, Ana Didović Pavičić and Robert Stanić

Abstract

In 1949, first intraocular lens (IOL) insertion after cataract surgery was performed by Sir Harold Ridley, in London. Only in the 1970s, the IOL insertion after cataract surgery began to be a standard procedure. The material the first IOL-s were composed of was polymethyl methacrylate (PMMA). The PMMA is a rigid material and the corneal incision had to be at least as big as the IOLs optic and it became its biggest disadvantage in the cataract surgery. The main goal of modern cataract surgery is as smallest incision possible, so the IOL-s had to be flexible and therefore foldable. This goal was achieved by improvements in the IOL design and materials that made them foldable. First foldable IOL-s were made of hydrogel but they were unstable and the development of the first silicone IOL-s overcame that problem. Foldable silicone IOL-s were first implanted in 1978 by Kai-yi Zhou. Foldable IOL's benefits are its compatibility with a small incision surgery that is self-sealing procedure and the possibility of insertion by a single-use applicators that made the surgery safer. In the future, we can expect some new, different and innovative approaches in the IOL design and materials.

1. Introduction

Intraocular lenses (IOL) are implanted in the eye in order to treat refractive errors produced by extraction of the lens as a standard procedure in cataract surgery.

IOL is designed and composed of optic—central part, and the haptics—side structures that keep the lens inside the capsular bag.

The first intraocular lens was inserted in 1949 after cataract surgery by Sir Harold Ridley in St Thomas Hospital in London [1]. The material the first IOLs were composed of was polymethyl methacrylate (PMMA). It was a rigid nonfoldable material making the placement of the IOL challenging [2]. In the 1970s, the new lighter posterior chamber IOLs were designed and had propylene haptics for better stabilization and ciliary sulcus fixation and the IOL insertion after cataract surgery began to be a standard procedure.

In the early 1980s, Epstein began to use lenses made of silicone with the intention to make them foldable. That way they could be inserted into the eye through the small incisions of 3 mm and less compared to 5–7 mm incisions needed for nonfoldable IOLs insertion [3, 4]. The practice of IOL implantation was revolutionized in 1984 when Thomas Mazzocco began folding and implanting the plate haptic silicone IOLs [5].

Current materials used for IOL optics are of two types—acrylic and silicone. Acrylic materials can be rigid (PMMA) and foldable made of hydrophobic acrylic materials (AcrySof - Alcon Laboratories, Sensar – Advanced Medical Optics – AMO) and hydrophilic acrylics (Centerflex, Akreos).

Each foldable acrylic lens design is made from a different copolymer acrylic with a different refractive index, glass transition temperature, water content, mechanical properties and other attributes.

Hydrophobic acrylic lenses and silicone lenses have very low water content (less than 1%). But there are hydrophobic acrylic materials with higher water content about 4% also available. Hydrophilic acrylic lenses are made from copolymers with higher water content ranging from 18 to 38%.

The first silicone material that was used in the industry of IOLs was polydimethylsiloxane, with refractive index of 1.41 while the new silicone materials have higher refractive indexes.

Refractive index in foldable acrylics is 1.47 or greater, and for silicone lenses is lower—1.41 and higher. Therefore acrylic lenses are thinner than silicone ones with the same refractive power.

2. Materials

2.1 Biocompatibility

The biocompatibility of a material is dependent of a biological response to a foreign body material and it depends on the design and the material of the implant. The material should be chemically inert, physically stable, noncarcinogenic, non-allergenic, capable of fabrication in the required form, and have no foreign body reaction [6]. Materials used in ophthalmology should also be optically transparent for long period of time, have a high resolving power or refractive index, and should block ultraviolet rays.

The reaction of lens epithelial cells and the capsule to IOL material and design is capsular biocompatibility. The uvea's reaction to the IOL is uveal biocompatibility [7]. During cataract surgery the blood-aqueous barrier is disrupted and proteins and cells are released in the aqueous humor. Proteins then adsorb on the IOL surface and this will influence subsequent cellular reactions on the IOL [8].

3. Glistenings

Glistenings are a phenomenon caused by penetration of aqueous humor into the IOL material causing vacuole formation in the IOLs optic [9].

Glistenings are fluid-filled microvacuoles that form within the IOL optic when the lens is in an aqueous environment. They can be observed with any type of IOL more often in association with hydrophobic acrylic lenses.

Factors that may influence the formation of glistenings include IOL material, manufacturing technique and packaging and also the associated conditions of the eye-glaucoma, conditions leading to breakdown of the blood-aqueous barrier and use of ocular medications.

Some theories refer glistenings as a cavitation within the IOL from slow moving hydrophilic impurities within the IOL. An osmotic pressure difference between the aqueous solution within a cavity and the external media in which the lens is immersed leads to growth of the cavity [10].

Glistening develop over time and indicate a dynamic process within the lens/eye system. Causes and long-term outcomes are not entirely clear [11].

Hydrophobic acrylic IOL have the highest degree of lens glistening in comparison to the silicone and the HSM-PMMA IOL 11.3–13.4 years after surgery. The HSM-PMMA IOL had almost no lens glistenings. Lens glistening do not interfere with the dioptric power of the hydrophobic acrylic lens IOL [12].

4. Hydrophobicity and hygroscopy

Hydrophobicity is a measure of material's tendency to separate itself from water. Every material has its measurable hydrophobicity that is graded using contact-angle measurements and it is a surface property [13–15]. It ranges from only a few degrees for almost perfectly hydrophilic surfaces, such as bare silica glass prepared with dangling hydroxyl groups [16] to almost 180° for super-hydrophobic surfaces [14].

Hydrophobicity is highly dependent of the material's chemistry since the oxygen–hydrogen bonds in water are highly polar. Partial electric charges on the atoms tend to be attracted to opposite charges. That way water dissolves salts and is attracted to materials that also have partially charged bonds. Polymers consist primarily of nonpolar carbon–carbon and carbon–hydrogen bonds, which is why they are not generally hydrophilic and is attracted to materials with partially charged bonds.

Hygroscopy explains a material's tendency to absorb and hold water. A highly hygroscopic material draws water into itself. In ophthalmology the hydrophobicity has been used to describe both the surface and interior of IOLs. The interaction of an IOL's surface with water is a measure of hydrophobicity and the ability of IOLs to draw water into their interior a hygroscopy.

5. Polymethyl methacrylate

The first IOL, implanted in 1949, was made of PMMA. There have been reports of original lenses implanted by Ridley remaining perfectly clear and centered for more than 28 years [3]. There were also reports of some spontaneous dislocations into the vitreous [5].

It is a rigid, nonfoldable material with less than 1% water content and therefore hydrophobic. PMMA IOLs are usually single pieced, large and therefore nowadays rarely used. They have a refractive index of 1.49 and usual optic diameter 5–7 mm. They are s too rigid to fold and therefore the lens cannot pass through the small incisions used phacoemulsification.

6. Silicone

Silicon IOLs were designed to allow implanting through the incision smaller than the optics diameter. Implantation of silicone IOLs was introduced in 1984 [17]. Silicone is a hydrophobic material of refractive index 1.41–1.46 and the optic diameter of 5.5–6.5 mm. Models are three-piece design with PMMA, polyvinyl difluoride (PVDF) and polyamide haptics. The problem with silicone is an abrupt opening in the anterior chamber following implantation which may cause rupture of the posterior capsule.

Silicone IOL-s suspected to favor bacterial adhesion and therefore having the higher risk of postoperative infections [18]. Silicone oil droplets adhere well to silicone IOL in patients with silicone oil tamponade used in retinal detachment or diabetic retinopathy surgery [19]. Therefore silicon IOL should not be implanted in highly myopic eyes in risk of retinal detachment.

Nowadays the silicone IOLs are less frequently used because they are not suitable for microincision cataract surgery (MICS).

There are also a light adjustable lens-two component silicone IOL where power is adjusted after implantation with UV-exposure in use [20, 21].

Glistenings can happen with silicone optics while the aqueous humor can penetrate the silicon material [12].

7. Hydrophobic foldable acrylic

Acrylic hydrophobic IOLs are modern foldable IOLs most widely used nowadays. They are designed of copolymers of acrylate and methacrylate derived from PMMA. The intention of the new design is to make the IOL foldable. They can be manipulated during the surgery and always turning back to its original shape [22] in a short period of time. First implanted IOL was in year 1993. Hydrophobic Foldable Acrylic can be of three piece and one piece design, with optic diameter 5.5–7 mm, and overall length 12–13 mm, transparent or colored—yellow. Refractive index can be 1.44–1.55.

Single and multi-piece hydrophobic IOLs can be implanted through small incision, not lover than 2.2 mm and have to be positioned properly since they have low self-centering ability. PCO is significantly lower than in PMMA IOLs but generally a bit higher for hydrophobic acrylic lenses compared with silicone [23].

They have higher incidence of photopsias than other acrylic IOLs because of high refractive index and low anterior curvatures and some of them develop glistenings since some are easily penetrated by aqueous humor but are not always clinically relevant unless when are dense or multifocal [24]. New materials of IOLs are prehydrated to equilibrium and will not accept further water, they are hydrophobic with the contact angle with water that of hydrophobic acrylic and are packaged in BSS to absorb the eventual water content before implantation [25].

8. Hydrophilic foldable acrylic

Hydrophilic foldable acrylic is a combination of hydroxyethylmethacrylate (polyHEMA) and hydrophilic acrylic monomer [26] material and it was introduced in 1980 with several modifications since. The IOLs made of this materials are usually single pieced and designed for capsular bag implantation. Refractive index of the material is 1.43, with water content ranging from 18 to 34% [27, 28].

They are soft, compressible with excellent biocompatibility for its hydrophilic surface. They can be implanted through a small incisions, lower than 2 mm and therefore ideal for MICS [29]. The folding of poly-HEMA chains depends on the level of hydration, and so the physical and optical properties of the polymer change as a function of water content. As the lenses hydrate, they absorb water and become soft and transparent.

The main disadvantage is the higher rate of optic opacification than in other materials and lower resistance for capsular bag contraction [30, 31].

9. The future of IOL s materials and designs

Considering the new knowledge and technological improvements and achievements, we can expect the new materials and designs of IOLs. In order to improve biocompatibility and refractive quality we expect some changes in shape of the IOLs (discoid, plate-lamellar, ball shaped) and therefore some novelties in implantation possibilities. The new neuro-ophthalmological knowledge and knowledge about adaptation and perception, industries based on robotic approach and innovations give us the right to expect some new and completely different IOLs in their shape, materials and functioning principle [32, 33]. In conclusion, in the future, we can expect some new, different and innovative approaches in the IOLs design and materials and refractive ophthalmology.

Author details

Samir Čanović[1*], Suzana Konjevoda[2], Ana Didović Pavičić[1] and Robert Stanić[3]

1 General Hospital - Zadar, Zadar, Croatia

2 General Hospital - Zadar, University of Zadar, Zadar, Croatia

3 Clinical Hospital Center Split, Split, Croatia

*Address all correspondence to: suzana.konjevoda@gmail.com

IntechOpen

© 2019 The Author(s). Licensee IntechOpen. This chapter is distributed under the terms of the Creative Commons Attribution License (http://creativecommons.org/licenses/by/3.0), which permits unrestricted use, distribution, and reproduction in any medium, provided the original work is properly cited.

References

[1] Ridley H. Intraocular acrylic lenses—Past, present and future. Transactions of the Ophthalmological Societies of the United Kingdom. 1964;**84**:5-14

[2] Apple DJ, Mamalis N, Loftfield K, Googe JM, Novak LC, Kavka-Van Norman D, et al. Complications of intraocular lenses. A historical and histopathological review. Survey of Ophthalmology. 1984;**29**:1-54

[3] Choyce DP. Discussion to Barraquer: Anterior chamber plastic lenses. Results of and conclusions from five years experience. Transactions of the Ophthalmological Societies of the United Kingdom. 1959;**79**:393-494

[4] Apple DJ, Escobar-Gomez M, Zaugg B, Kleinmann G, Borkenstein AF. Modern cataract surgery: Unfinished business and unanswered questions. Survey of Ophthalmology. 2011;**56**:S3-S53

[5] Epstein E. History of intraocular lens implant surgery. In: Mazzocico TRRG, Epstein E, editors. Soft Implant Lenses in Cataract Surgery. Thorofare, NJ: Slock Inc; 1986

[6] Scales J. Discussion on metals and synthetic materials in relation to tissues; tissue reactions to synthetic materials. Proceedings of the Royal Society of Medicine. 1953;**46**:647-652

[7] Werner L. Biocompatibility of intraocular lens materials. Current Opinion in Ophthalmology. 2008;**19**:41-49. Review

[8] Abela-Formanek C, Amon M, Schild G, Schauersberger J, Heinze G, Kruger A. Uveal and capsular biocompatibility of hydrophilic acrylic, hydrophobic acrylic, and silicone intraocular lenses. Journal of Cataract and Refractive Surgery. 2002;**28**:50-61

[9] Michelson J, Werner L, Ollerton A, Leishman L, Bodnar Z. Light scattering and light transmittance in intraocular lenses explanted because of optic opacification. Journal of Cataract and Refractive Surgery. 2012;**38**:1476-1485

[10] Saylor DM, Coleman Richardson D, Dair BJ, Pollack SK. Osmotic cavitation of elastomeric intraocular lenses. Acta Biomaterialia. 2010;**6**:1090-1098

[11] Miyata A, Suzuki K, Boku C, Kinohira Y, Aramaki T, Ando M, et al. Glistening particles on the implanted acrylic intraocular lens

[12] Rønbeck M, Behndig A, Taube M, Koivula A, Kugelberg M. Comparison of glistenings in intraocular lenses with three different materials: 12-year follow-up. Acta Ophthalmologica. 2013;**91**:66-70

[13] Scatena LF, Brown MG, Richmond GL. Water at hydrophobic surfaces: Weak hydrogen bonding and strong orientation effects. Science. 2001;**292**:908-912

[14] Ma M, Hill RM. Superhydrophobic surfaces. Current Opinion in Colloid & Interface Science. 2006;**11**:193-202

[15] Cao L, Hu H-H, Gao D. Design and fabrication of microtextures for inducing a superhydrophobic behavior on hydrophilic materials. Langmuir. 2007;**23**:4310-4314

[16] Sugimura H, Ushiyama K, Hozumi A, Takai O. Micropatterning of alkyl- and fluoroalkylsilane selfassembled monolayers using vacuum ultraviolet light. Langmuir. 2000;**16**:885-888

[17] Mazzocco TR, Rajacich GM, Epstein E. Soft implant lenses in cataract surgery. Thorofare: Slack; 1986

[18] Baillif S, Ecochard R, Hartmann D, Freney J, Kodjikian L. Intraocular lens

and cataract surgery: Comparison between bacterial adhesion and risk of postoperative endophthalmitis according to intraocular lens biomaterial (in French). Journal Français d'Ophtalmologie. 2009;**32**:515-528

[19] Bartz-Schmidt KU, Konen W, Esser P, Walter P, Heimann K. Intraocular silicone lenses and silicone oil (in German). Klinische Monatsblätter für Augenheilkunde. 1995;**207**:162-166

[20] von Mohrenfels CW, Salgado J, Kho-ramnia R, Maier M, Lohmann CP. Clinical results with the light adjustable intraocular lens after cataract surgery. Journal of Refractive Surgery. 2010;**26**:314-320

[21] Hengerer FH, Hütz WW, Dick HB, Conrad-Hengerer I. Combined correction of axial hyperopia and astigmatism using the light adjustable intraocular lens. Ophthalmology. 2011;**118**:1236-1241

[22] Oshika T, Shiokawa Y. Effect of folding on the optical quality of soft acrylic intraocular lenses. Journal of Cataract and Refractive Surgery. 2002;**28**:1141-1152

[23] Abela-Formanek C, Amon M, Schauersberger J, Kruger A, Nepp J, Schild G. Results of hydrophilic acrylic, hydrophobicacrylic, and silicone intraocular lenses in uveiticeyes with cataract: Comparison to a control group. Journal of Cataract & Refractive Surgery. 1996;**22**(Suppl 2):1360-1364

[24] Miura M, Osako M, Elsner AE, Kajizuka H, Yamada K, Usui M. Birefringence of intraocular lenses. Journal of Cataract and Refractive Surgery. 2004;**30**:1549-1555

[25] Ollerton A, Werner L, Fuller SR, Kavoussi SC, McIntyre JS, Mamalis N. Evaluation of a new single-piece 4% water content hydrophobic acrylic intraocular lens in the rabbit model. Journal of Cataract and Refractive Surgery. 2012;**38**:1827-1832

[26] Chehade M, Elder MJ. Intraocular lens materials and styles: A review. Australian and New Zealand Journal of Ophthalmology. 1997;**25**:255-263

[27] Allarakhia L, Knoll RL, Lindstrom RL. Soft intraocular lenses. Journal of Cataract and Refractive Surgery. 1987;**13**:607-620

[28] Tehrani M, Dick HB, Wolters B, Pakula T, Wolf E. Material properties of various intraocular lenses in an experimental study. Ophthalmologica. 2004;**218**:57-63

[29] Kohnen T, Klaproth OK. Intraocular lenses for microincisional cataract surgery (in German). Der Ophthalmologe. 2010;**107**:127-135

[30] Hazra S, Palui H, Vemuganti GK. Comparison of design of intraocular lens versus the material for PCO prevention. International Journal of Ophthalmology. 2012;**5**:59-63

[31] Apple DJ, Werner L. Complications of cataract and refractive surgery: A clinicopathological documentation. Transactions of the American Ophthalmological Society. 2001;**99**:95-109

[32] Andrews T. Stereoscopic depth perception during binocular rivalry. Frontiers in Human Neuroscience. 2011;**5**:99

[33] Jiang B, Yang J, Lv Z, Song H. Wearable vision assistance system based on binocular sensors for visually impaired users. IEEE Internet of Things Journal. 2019;**6**(2):1375-1383

Section 2

Aberration and Astigmatism Correction with Intraocular Lens

Chapter 3

Aberration Correction with Aspheric Intraocular Lenses

Timo Eppig, Jens Schrecker, Arthur Messner and Achim Langenbucher

Abstract

The shape of the normal human cornea induces positive spherical aberration (SA) which causes image blur. In the young phakic eye, the crystalline lens compensates for a certain amount of this corneal aberration. However, the compensation slowly decreases with the aging lens and is fully lost after cataract extraction and implantation of a standard intraocular lens (IOL). Conventional spherical IOLs add their intrinsic positive SA to the positive SA of the cornea increasing the image blur. As a useful side effect, this also increases the depth of focus—often referred to as pseudo-accommodation. Aspheric intraocular lenses have been introduced to be either neutral to SA or to compensate for a certain amount of corneal SA. A customized correction for the individual eye seems to be the most promising solution for tailored correction of SA. In this chapter we will provide detailed information on the various concepts of aspheric intraocular lenses to elucidate that the term "aspheric intraocular lens" is being used for a large amount of different lens designs.

Keywords: spherical aberration, aspheric surface, customized intraocular lens, decentration, tilt

1. Introduction

The disease pattern of cataract comprises pathologic conditions of the human eye resulting from an opacification of the crystalline lens. The most frequent causes for the development of cataract are age-related transformation processes. Although research on pharmacologic treatment of cataract has been in focus for many years, the surgical extraction of the cloudy crystalline lens and implantation of an artificial intraocular lens (IOL)—referred to as cataract surgery—represent the only available treatment. Cataract surgery is one of the most frequently performed surgical procedures with several million surgeries being performed worldwide each year.

First IOL developments were primarily targeted on biocompatible materials and new fixation techniques rather than on correction of ocular aberrations other than defocus and astigmatism. First lens implants were made from polymethyl methacrylate, therefore being rigid and requiring large incisions for implantation. Furthermore, the optimum site of implantation (anterior chamber, iris, ciliary sulcus, or capsular bag) still had to be found, and adequate haptics for proper fixation had to be developed. Surgical results were therefore less predictable [1, 2].

In the early 1980s, foldable silicone materials and later acrylic materials allowed implantation through smaller ports and therefore caused less damage to the corneal structure allowing a faster rehabilitation. This finally facilitated ambulant cataract surgery. In the following years, the capsular bag was identified as the optimum position for an IOLs, and the development of new lens power calculation formulas dramatically increased the predictability of the refractive outcome [1].

2. Aspheric lenses

With the improvement in IOL power calculation, the goal of cataract surgery became predictable; the focus of cataract surgery shifted from "restoration of vision" to "refractive surgery." Manufacturers started optimizing the IOL optic from an equiconvex spherical lens design to different aspheric surface profiles and finally multifocal and free-form surface designs. The buzzword of those days was "spherical aberration" (SA) which should be eliminated to improve contrast sensitivity and visual acuity. Spherical aberration is one of the monochromatic aberrations that is caused by the difference in focal length (or optical power) for varying aperture diameter of a lens. For positive spherical aberration, the optical power increases from the lens center to the periphery, and rays far from the optical axis will intersect the optical axis in front of the paraxial focus (**Figure 1**).

Any spherical optical surface causes SA. To achieve an equal distribution of optical power across the lens diameter, the optical surfaces have to be tailored accordingly. SA can only be reduced by varying the spherical radii of curvature of anterior and posterior surface yielding a so called best-form lens, but it cannot be eliminated. This can be achieved by implementing aspheric surfaces. There are basically two types of aspheric surfaces that have been described in the literature, the first one is referred to as "continuous asphere" and can be described by the formula

$$z = \frac{\frac{1}{r} \cdot \rho^2}{1 + \sqrt{1 - (1-Q) \cdot \frac{1}{r^2} \rho^2}} + \sum_{n=1}^{n=8} a_{2n} \cdot \rho^{2n} + X \qquad (1)$$

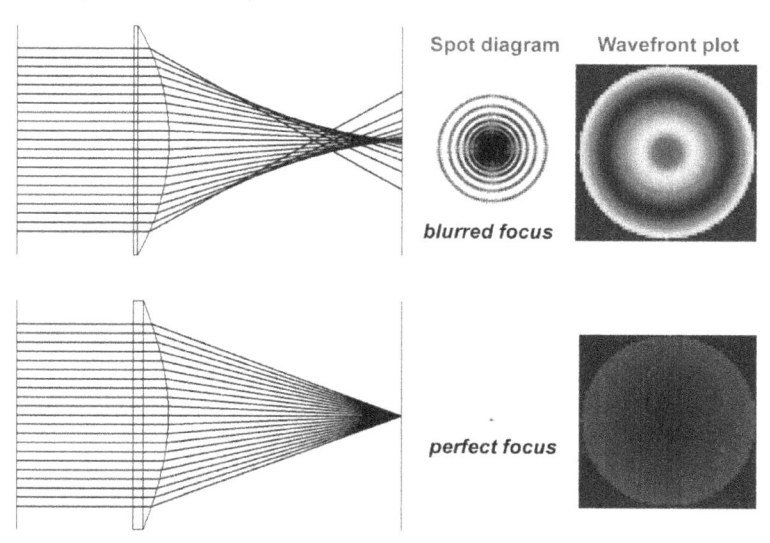

Figure 1.
Rays focused by a lens with positive spherical aberration (top) compared to a lens without spherical aberration (bottom) [4].

where z is the height of the surface from the apex (= 0 mm), r is the radius of curvature, and ρ is the radial coordinate from the center to the periphery. Q is called "asphericity" [3], and a_{2n} are higher-order aspheric coefficients. X is a placeholder for additional polynomials, such as Zernike polynomials, which can be used to define additional surface shapes. From this equation numerous aspheric surface profiles can be generated (**Figure 2**), and most of current aspheric intraocular lens designs are based on the formula above. Equation (1) can be expanded to represent toric and biconic surfaces as well. The asphericity Q is identical to the conic constant κ (often used in optical design software) and can be transformed from other shape definitions for the aspheric surface such as the eccentricity e or the index of eccentricity e^2 [3]:

$$Q = -e^2 \qquad (2)$$

The second type of aspherical surfaces, called "zonal asphere," is constructed from a set of annular rings with varying radius of curvature and asphericity. For a detailed description of these surfaces, please refer to the literature [5, 6].

By modulating radius of curvature, asphericity, and aspheric coefficients, the SA induced by the surface can be customized. Additional polynomials can be added on top to create non-rotationally symmetric aspheric surfaces to compensate for higher-order errors such as coma or trefoil. For example, one alternate way to compensate for spherical aberration would be to modulate the aspherical surface with a linear combination of Zernike polynomials representing various orders of spherical aberration:

$$X = C_{11} \cdot Z_4^0 + C_{22} \cdot Z_6^0 + C_{37} \cdot Z_8^0 + \cdots \qquad (3)$$

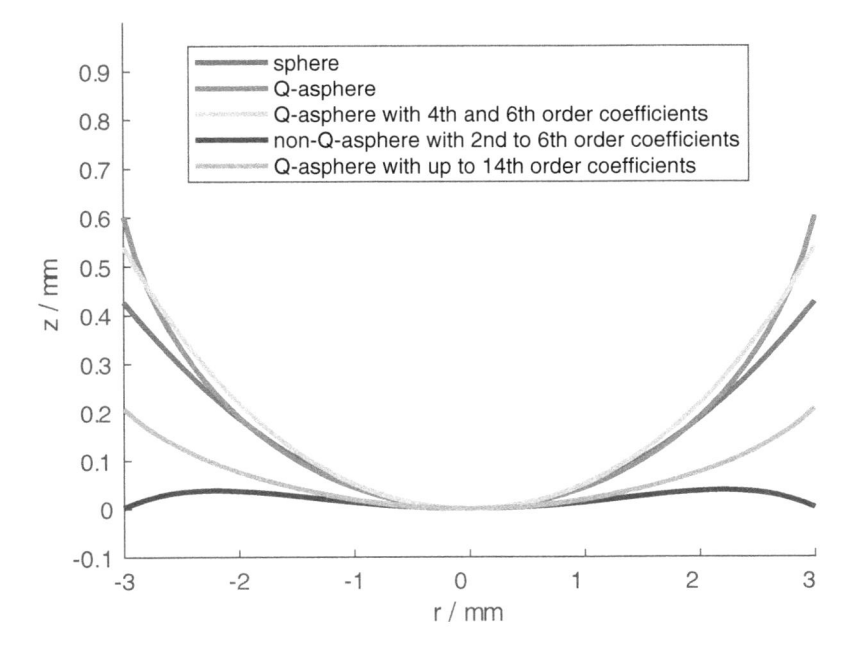

Figure 2.
Variation of optical surface section with increasing number of coefficients. z is the elevation relative to the surface apex. All curves are derived from intraocular lens designs for an average power (20 to 22 D) lens.

3. Corneal spherical aberration

As mentioned above, the average human cornea induces a significant portion of positive SA, which is typically being described by the Zernike coefficient Z_4^0 (spherical aberration) on a diameter of 6.0 mm at corneal plane. The amount of SA can be calculated from the corneal surface shape by optical ray tracing. A method to do so was described by Norrby et al. providing a reference value for the Liou-Brennan model eye [7, 8]. Calossi provided an overview of SA values for a limited set of variables [3].

Depending on the underlying database, various authors reported different values for the average corneal SA. Holladay et al. reported that the average SA of the human cornea is about +0.27 ± 0.20 µm (value misprinted in the original publication [9] and corrected by Norrby et al. [7]). Similar values were found by Beiko and Haigis (+0.274 ± 0.089 µm) [10]. The widely spread Liou-Brennan model eye provides about +0.258 µm of spherical aberration being close to the reported average clinical values [7, 8]. De Sanctis et al. found higher values in their patients (+0.328 ± 0.132 µm) [11], while Shimozono et al. found lower values (0.203 ± 0.100 µm) [12].

4. Correction of spherical aberration with IOLs

Aberration correction could be best described as a superposition of wave fronts as outlined in **Figure 3**.

During cataract surgery the corneal SA is typically increased by the likewise positive spherical aberration of a spherical IOL. Therefore, lens designers at first created the "aberration-free" or "aberration-neutral" lens concept, a lens design that was meant to eliminate its intrinsic spherical aberration and thus being neutral to the eye's overall SA [13]. However, the amount of SA is highly depending on the vergence of the incident rays. Therefore, there are differences in the design of "aberration-neutral" lenses: some of them are designed to be neutral to SA in a collimated beam, e.g., a beam as such could be used in measurement instrumentation. Others are designed to be neutral to SA behind some generic model cornea (in a converging beam). Both of them will exhibit a considerable amount of SA when implanted in a real eye; the first will provide a small correction for SA, while the latter may provide

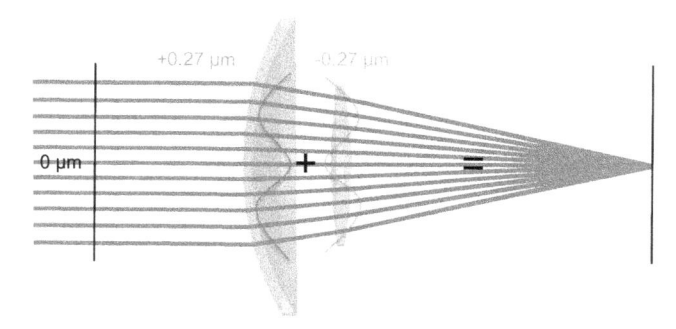

Figure 3.
Simplified sketch of the principle of aberration correction: An impinging plane wave front (collimated beam) is refracted by the cornea and affected by spherical aberration (red); the intraocular lens (yellow) compensates for the same amount of spherical aberration (green) resulting in a perfect wave front at the focus plane. Note: The plotted wave fronts do not account for the defocus.

Manufacturer	Product	SA correction
Johnson & Johnson Vision, Groningen, The Netherlands	TECNIS	−0.27 µm [9]
HOYA, Nagoya, Japan	Vivinex XC1	−0.18 µm [17, 18]
Carl Zeiss Meditec, Berlin, Germany	CT ASPHINA 509MP	−0.18 µm [18]
Alcon Laboratories, Forth Worth, TX, USA	AcrySof IQ SN60WF	−0.17 µm [17]
Bausch + Lomb, Rochester, NY, USA	EyeCee One	−0.14 µm [18]
	Quatrix Evolutive	−0.1 µm [18]
PhysIOL, Liege, Belgium	PODeye	−0.11 µm [18]
Kowa Pharmaceuticals, Düsseldorf, Germany	AvanSee	−0.04 [18]

Table 1.
List of selected intraocular lens models providing correction of spherical aberration.

negligible change to the corneal SA. When being analyzed on an optical bench (in a collimated beam), both lenses will show the opposite characteristics [4].

Aberration-correcting designs evolved subsequently, providing compensation to a fixed amount of corneal SA. One of the first aberration-correcting lenses was presented by Holladay et al. providing a correction of −0.27 µm and thus targeting on the average SA found in human eyes [9].

Today, surgeons may choose from a variety of aspheric IOLs with different amount of compensation for SA (**Table 1**). Theoretically, one could choose the IOL providing the optimum correction for an eye. This would require preoperative examination of corneal topography and analysis of corneal aberrations. Diagnostic instrumentation for the anterior segment such as the Pentacam (Oculus Optikgeräte GmbH, Wetzlar, Germany) or the CASIA2 (Tomey Corp., Nagoya, Japan) allow direct readout of the SA amount over 6 mm diameter. The SA value calculated from corneal tomographic data could then be used to select an IOL model that provides best correction. Still, since the range of IOLs with different SA corrections is limited, not every eye could be supplied with optimum correction. Clinical results with this "selection method" are controversial but indicate the potential for improvement [14–16]. Piers et al. found that contrast sensitivity peaks with 0 µm of SA [17]. On the contrary, other investigators found that a residual SA of about +0.1 µm may be beneficial for visual performance [18–20]. Manzanera and Artal argued that changes in SA between −0.17 and + 0.2 µm are merely noticeable by patients [21]. This may be an explanation why the differences in visual performance between aberration-free and aberration-correcting lenses are usually small.

The next logical step is a compensation procedure based on the true individual SA, rather than on average values. Wang et al. found that not only SA should be considered but the full spectrum of corneal aberrations [22–24]. Especially eyes with high amounts of spherical aberration such as eyes after laser refractive surgery or eyes with forme fruste keratoconus could benefit more from customized correction of SA [22, 23, 25] than normal eyes, if centration of the implant can be kept within strict limits. Therefore, an optimum solution could be the customization of intraocular lenses [26, 27]. Several researchers provided theoretical basics and theoretical results showing the potential of customized intraocular lenses [28–31]. The design process of such IOLs requires the implementation of customized model eyes based on biometric data and the use of ray tracing technology [28, 32–36]. The first clinical results with this method have recently been published showing promising results [37].

5. Limitations of aberration-correcting lenses

A major limitation for the selection of the appropriate IOL is the accuracy and repeatability of the preoperative corneal topography. The calculation of corneal SA requires highest precision of corneal topography in the periphery, since the difference in elevation between an aspheric corneal surface and a spherical surface is only some microns (**Figure 4**). Schröder et al. investigated the measurement repeatability and precision of several corneal topographers and tomographers and found that the repeatability of these devices is decreasing from the center to the periphery and may not be sufficient to detect small changes in corneal asphericity [38].

Another limitation arises from the concept of aberration correction itself. As outlined in **Figure 3**, the method requires the alignment of the IOL in relation to the cornea to be as perfect as possible. But even if an ideal positioning of the IOL is achieved intraoperatively, the risk of decentration or tilt remains in the postoperative course.

Altmann et al., Eppig et al., and others analyzed the effects of decentration and tilt of spherical and aspherical IOLs on the image quality and found that it is more affected by decentration than by tilt and that the susceptibility of lens misalignment increases with the amount of SA to be corrected [9, 39–46]. Some authors defined that a range of decentration within a SA-correcting IOL would perform better or equal than a standard spherical IOL. This range was reported to be between 0.0 and 0.3–0.8 mm, depending on the design of the lens and simulation conditions [9, 40–42]. In a previous publication, we summarized the data on the IOL decentration from various sources and found that the clinically observed decentration is between 0 and 1 mm but most frequently about 0.3 mm [33, 40, 47–56]. Others showed that there is a tendency for IOLs decentering and tilting into nasal direction with mirror symmetry between both eyes [51].

Gillner et al. showed in a previous publication that IOL designs with a more conservative correction of SA may provide a larger range of tolerance to decentration [41]. Examples thereof are the ZO/ASPHINA design (Carl Zeiss Meditec AG, Berlin, Germany) and the Aspheric Balanced Curve Design (ABCD) (Hoya Corporation, Tokyo, Japan). Both designs are based on higher-order

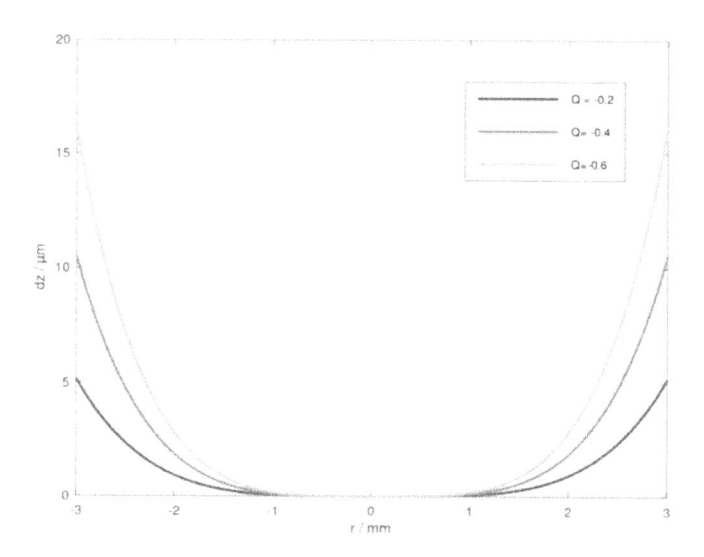

Figure 4.
Difference in corneal elevation for three surfaces with R = 7.77 mm radius of curvature and several values of Q compared to a sphere.

aspherics including coefficients a_4 and higher (see Eq. 1) and were specifically designed considering some reasonable amount of IOL decentration. The effect of decentration on image performance of some selected IOL designs is shown in **Figures 5** and **6**. The graphs exhibit a drop of the image quality with aspheric lenses below the image quality of a spherical IOL when decentration exceeds 0.4 and 0.3 mm, respectively.

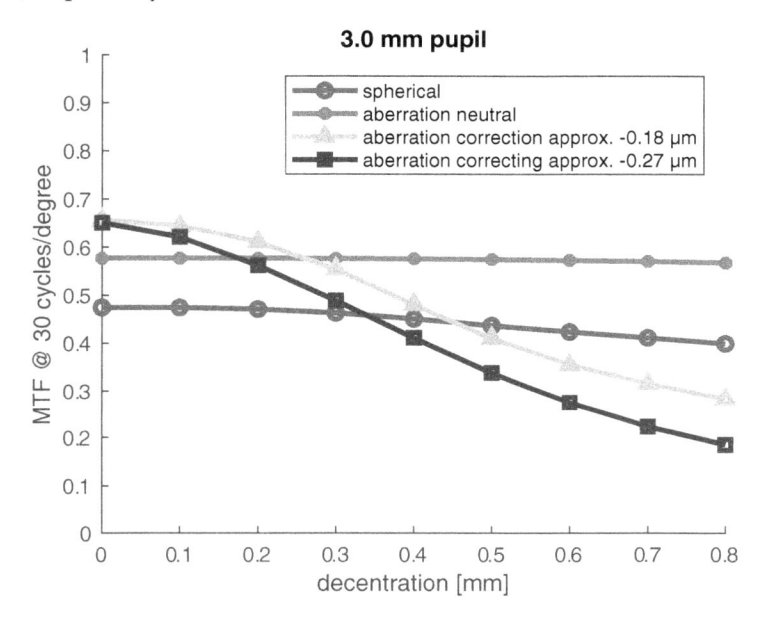

Figure 5.
Simulation of modulation transfer function at 30 cycles per degree for four different intraocular lenses and a pupil diameter of 3.0 mm in the Liou-Brennan model eye as a function of decentration [40, 41, 57].

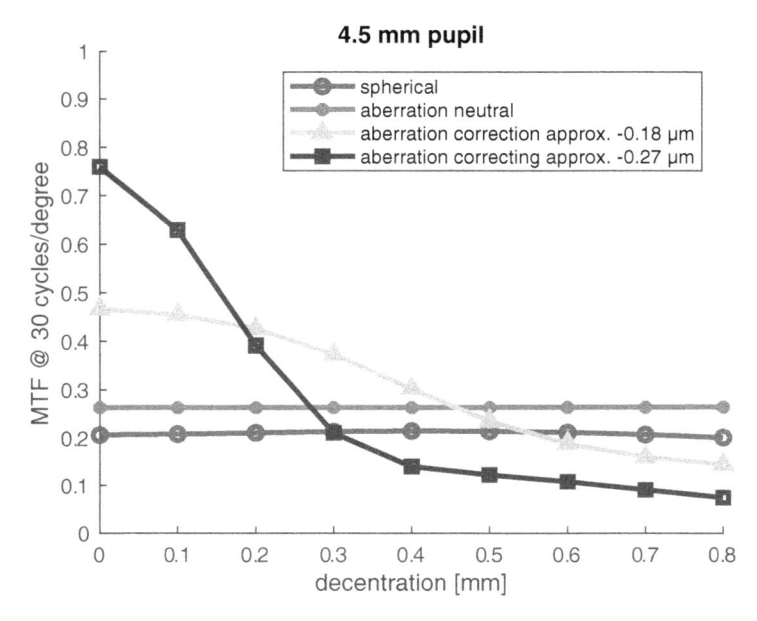

Figure 6.
Simulation of modulation transfer function at 30 cycles per degree for four different intraocular lenses and a pupil diameter of 4.5 mm in the Liou-Brennan model eye as a function of decentration [40, 41].

6. Conclusions

Correcting the spherical aberration of the cornea by intraocular lenses may improve the visual outcome compared to standard spherical lenses. Especially patients with high aberrations after corneal refractive surgery may benefit from a reduction of the overall aberrations. However, the prospects for a 100% correction of SA or aiming to a residual SA of +0.1 µm are limited with respect to an ideal and stable IOL. Therefore, any generic or customized IOL concept pursuing an aberration correction of aberrations, such as astigmatism, spherical aberration, coma, etc. must be designed with a tolerance according to the average expected misalignment in normal eyes (approximately 0–0.3 mm decentration and 0–3 degrees of tilt) [40, 57]. Consequently, this likewise limits the correctability of some higher-order aberrations. Eyes after corneal refractive surgery usually show very high values of SA and require special attention in the planning of cataract surgery. While eyes after myopic refractive procedures might benefit from a negative SA IOL [22], eyes after hyperopic refractive procedures often show high-negative SA and would require an IOL with positive SA for compensation [23]. Due to the high variability of SA in cataract patients, the "one-size-fits-all" approach may only provide optimum correction for a small amount of patients. Therefore, customized intraocular lenses tailored to correct for the individual spherical aberration may provide a better solution for a wide range of patients.

Author details

Timo Eppig[1,2]*, Jens Schrecker[3], Arthur Messner[1] and Achim Langenbucher[2]

1 AMIPLANT GmbH, Schnaittach, Germany

2 Institute of Experimental Ophthalmology, Saarland University, Homburg, Germany

3 Department of Ophthalmology, Rudolf-Virchow-Klinikum, Glauchau, Germany

*Address all correspondence to: timo.eppig@uks.eu

IntechOpen

© 2019 The Author(s). Licensee IntechOpen. This chapter is distributed under the terms of the Creative Commons Attribution License (http://creativecommons.org/licenses/by/3.0), which permits unrestricted use, distribution, and reproduction in any medium, provided the original work is properly cited.

References

[1] Auffarth GU, Apple DJ. Zur Entwicklungsgeschichte der Intraokularlinsen. Der Ophthalmologe. 2001;98(11):1017-1028

[2] Apple DJ. Sir Harold Ridley and his Fight for Sight: He Changed the World so that we May Better See it. 10th ed. Thorofare, NJ, USA: Slack Inc.; 2006

[3] Calossi A. Corneal asphericity and spherical aberration. Journal of Refractive Surgery. 2007;23(5):505-514

[4] Eppig T, Schröder S, Schrecker J, et al. Do aberration neutral intraocular lens designs effectively induce no spherical aberration? In: 35th Congress of the European Society of Cataract and Refractive Surgery. Lisbon 2017. Available from: https://www.escrs.org/abstracts/details.asp?confid=24&sessid=1078&type=poster&paperid=28779 [Accessed: 09 August 2019]

[5] Smith G, Atchison DA. Construction, specification, and mathematical description of aspheric surfaces. American Journal of Optometry and Physiological Optics. 1983;60(3):216-223

[6] Atchison DA. Design of aspheric intraocular lenses. Ophthalmic and Physiological Optics. 1991;11(2):137-146

[7] Norrby S, Piers P, Campbell C, et al. Model eyes for evaluation of intraocular lenses. Applied Optics. 2007;46(26):6595-6605

[8] Liou H-L, Brennan NA. Anatomically accurate, finite model eye for optical modeling. Journal of the Optical Society of America. A. 1997;14(8):1684-1695

[9] Holladay JT, Piers PA, Koranyi G, et al. A new intraocular lens design to reduce spherical aberration of pseudophakic eyes. Journal of Refractive Surgery. 2002;18(6):683-691

[10] Beiko GHH, Haigis W, Steinmueller A. Distribution of corneal spherical aberration in a comprehensive ophthalmology practice and whether keratometry can predict aberration values. Journal of Cataract and Refractive Surgery. 2007;33(5):848-858

[11] de Sanctis U, Vinai L, Bartoli E, et al. Total spherical aberration of the cornea in patients with cataract. Optometry and Vision Science. 2014;91(10):1251-1258

[12] Shimozono M, Uemura A, Hirami Y, et al. Corneal spherical aberration of eyes with cataract in a Japanese population. Journal of Refractive Surgery. 2010;26(6):457-459

[13] Langenbucher A, Schröder S, Cayless A, et al. Aberration-free intraocular lenses—what does this really mean? Zeitschrift für Medizinische Physik. 2017;27(3):255-259

[14] Nochez Y, Favard A, Majzoub S, et al. Measurement of corneal aberrations for customisation of intraocular lens asphericity: Impact on quality of vision after micro-incision cataract surgery. The British Journal of Ophthalmology. 2010;94(4):440-444

[15] Tan Q-Q, Lin J, Tian J, et al. Objective optical quality in eyes with customized selection of aspheric intraocular lens implantation. BMC Ophthalmology. 2019;19(1):152

[16] Jia L-X, Li Z-H. Clinical study of customized aspherical intraocular lens implants. International Journal of Ophthalmology. 2014;7(5):816-821

[17] Piers PA, Manzanera S, Prieto PM, et al. Use of adaptive optics to determine the optimal ocular spherical aberration. Journal of Cataract and Refractive Surgery. 2007;33(10):1721-1726

[18] Nochez Y, Majzoub S, Pisella P-J. Effect of residual ocular spherical aberration on objective and subjective quality of vision in pseudophakic eyes. Journal of Cataract and Refractive Surgery. 2011;**37**(6):1076-1081

[19] Werner JS, Elliott SL, Choi SS, et al. Spherical aberration yielding optimum visual performance: Evaluation of intraocular lenses using adaptive optics simulation. Journal of Cataract and Refractive Surgery. 2009;**35**(7):1229-1233

[20] Ferrer-Blasco T. Effect of partial and full correction of corneal spherical aberration on visual acuity and contrast sensitivity. Journal of Cataract and Refractive Surgery. 2009;**35**(5):949-951

[21] Manzanera S, Artal P. Minimum change in spherical aberration that can be perceived. Biomedical Optics Express. 2016;**7**(9):3471-3477

[22] Wang L, Pitcher JD, Weikert MP, et al. Custom selection of aspheric intraocular lenses after wavefront-guided myopic photorefractive keratectomy. Journal of Cataract and Refractive Surgery. 2010;**36**(1):73-81

[23] Wang L, Shoukfeh O, Koch DD. Custom selection of aspheric intraocular lens in eyes with previous hyperopic corneal surgery. Journal of Cataract and Refractive Surgery. 2015;**41**(12):2652-2663

[24] Koch DD, Wang L. Custom optimization of intraocular lens asphericity. Transactions of the American Ophthalmological Society. 2007;**105**:36-41; discussion 41-42

[25] Schröder S, Eppig T, Liu W, et al. Keratoconic eyes with stable corneal tomography could benefit more from custom intraocular lens design than normal eyes. Scientific Reports. 2019;**9**(1):3479

[26] Altmann GE. Wavefront-customized intraocular lenses. Current Opinion in Ophthalmology. 2004;**15**(4):358-364

[27] Beiko GHH. Personalized correction of spherical aberration in cataract surgery. Journal of Cataract and Refractive Surgery. 2007;**33**(8):1455-1460

[28] Einighammer J, Oltrup T, Feudner E, et al. Customized aspheric intraocular lenses calculated with real ray tracing. Journal of Cataract and Refractive Surgery. 2009;**35**(11):1984-1994

[29] Langenbucher A, Eppig T, Seitz B, et al. Customized aspheric IOL design by raytracing through the eye containing quadric surfaces. Current Eye Research. 2011;**36**(7):637-646

[30] Langenbucher A, Janunts E, Seitz B, et al. Theoretical image performance with customized aspheric and spherical IOLs - when do we get a benefit from customized aspheric design? Zeitschrift für Medizinische Physik. 2014;**24**(2):94-103

[31] Piers PA, Weeber HA, Artal P, et al. Theoretical comparison of aberration-correcting customized and aspheric intraocular lenses. Journal of Refractive Surgery. 2007;**23**(4):374-384

[32] Zhu Z, Janunts E, Eppig T, et al. Tomography-based customized IOL calculation model. Current Eye Research. 2011;**36**(6):579-589

[33] Rosales P, Marcos S. Customized computer models of eyes with intraocular lenses. Optics Express. 2007;**15**(5):2204-2218

[34] Ortiz S, Pérez-Merino P, Durán S, et al. Full OCT anterior segment biometry: An application in cataract surgery. Biomedical Optics Express. 2013;**4**(3):387-396

[35] Sun M, Pérez-Merino P, Martinez-Enriquez E, et al. Full 3-D OCT-based pseudophakic custom computer eye model. Biomedical Optics Express. 2016; 7(3):1074-1088

[36] Preussner P-R, Wahl J, Lahdo H, et al. Ray tracing for intraocular lens calculation. Journal of Cataract and Refractive Surgery. 2002;28(8): 1412-1419

[37] Schrecker J, Langenbucher A, Seitz B, et al. First results with a new intraocular lens design for the individual correction of spherical aberration. Journal of Cataract and Refractive Surgery. 2018;44(10):1211-1219

[38] Schröder S, Mäurer S, Eppig T, et al. Comparison of corneal tomography: Repeatability, precision, misalignment, mean elevation, and mean pachymetry. Current Eye Research. 2018;43(6): 709-716

[39] Altmann GE, Nichamin LD, Lane SS, et al. Optical performance of 3 intraocular lens designs in the presence of decentration. Journal of Cataract and Refractive Surgery. 2005;31(3):574-585

[40] Eppig T, Scholz K, Löffler A, et al. Effect of decentration and tilt on the image quality of aspheric intraocular lens designs in a model eye. Journal of Cataract and Refractive Surgery. 2009; 35(6):1091-1100

[41] Gillner M, Langenbucher A, Eppig T. Untersuchung der theoretischen Abbildungsqualität asphärischer Intraokularlinsen bei Dezentrierung. Hoya AF-1 iMics1 und Zeiss ASPHINA(TM) (Invent ZO). Der Ophthalmologe. 2012;109(3):263-270

[42] Pieh S, Fiala W, Malz A, et al. In vitro strehl ratios with spherical, aberration-free, average, and customized spherical aberration-correcting intraocular lenses. Investigative Ophthalmology and Visual Science. 2009;50(3):1264-1270

[43] Ortiz C, Esteve-Taboada JJ, Belda-Salmerón L, et al. Effect of decentration on the optical quality of two intraocular lenses. Optometry and Vision Science. 2016;93(12):1552-1559

[44] Dietze HH, Cox MJ. Limitations of correcting spherical aberration with aspheric intraocular lenses. Journal of Refractive Surgery. 2005;21(5):S541-S546

[45] Turuwhenua J. A theoretical study of intraocular lens tilt and decentration on perceptual image quality. Ophthalmic and Physiological Optics. 2005;25(6):556-567

[46] Pérez-Merino P, Marcos S. Effect of intraocular lens decentration on image quality tested in a custom model eye. Journal of Cataract and Refractive Surgery. 2018;44(7):889-896

[47] Kim JS, Shyn KH. Biometry of 3 types of intraocular lenses using Scheimpflug photography. Journal of Cataract and Refractive Surgery. 2001; 27(4):533-536

[48] Taketani F, Matuura T, Yukawa E, et al. Influence of intraocular lens tilt and decentration on wavefront aberrations. Journal of Cataract and Refractive Surgery. 2004;30(10): 2158-2162

[49] Baumeister M, Neidhardt B, Strobel J, et al. Tilt and decentration of three-piece foldable high-refractive silicone and hydrophobic acrylic intraocular lenses with 6-mm optics in an intraindividual comparison. American Journal of Ophthalmology. 2005;140(6):1051-1058

[50] Mutlu FM, Erdurman C, Sobaci G, et al. Comparison of tilt and decentration of 1-piece and 3-piece hydrophobic acrylic intraocular lenses.

Journal of Cataract and Refractive Surgery. 2005;**31**(2):343-347

[51] de Castro A, Rosales P, Marcos S. Tilt and decentration of intraocular lenses in vivo from Purkinje and Scheimpflug imaging. Validation study. Journal of Cataract and Refractive Surgery. 2007;**33**(3):418-429

[52] Mester U, Heinen S, Kaymak H. Klinische Ergebnisse unter besonderer Berücksichtigung von Dezentrierung und Verkippung der asphärischen Intraokularlinse FY-60AD. Der Ophthalmologe. 2010;**107**(9):831-836

[53] Choi SK, Kim JH, Lee D, et al. IOL tilt and decentration. Ophthalmology. 2010;**117**(9):1862, 1862.e1-1862, 1862.e4

[54] Sauer T, Mester U. Tilt and decentration of an intraocular lens implanted in the ciliary sulcus after capsular bag defect during cataract surgery. Graefe's Archive for Clinical and Experimental Ophthalmology. 2013;**251**(1):89-93

[55] Wang X, Dong J, Wang X, et al. IOL tilt and decentration estimation from 3 dimensional reconstruction of OCT image. PLoS One. 2013;**8**(3):e59109

[56] Findl O, Hirnschall N, Nishi Y, et al. Capsular bag performance of a hydrophobic acrylic 1-piece intraocular lens. Journal of Cataract and Refractive Surgery. 2015;**41**(1):90-97

[57] Ale JB. Intraocular lens tilt and decentration: A concern for contemporary IOL designs. Nepalese Journal of Ophthalmology. 2011;**3**(1):68-77

Chapter 4

Toric Intraocular Lenses

Zequan Xu

Abstract

This chapter described a short history about the toric intraocular lenses (IOLs) and then discussed some interesting topics such as the measurement of (front and posterior) corneal astigmatism and surgically induced astigmatism; the manual marking techniques and image-guided systems and intraoperative aberrometry-based methods; the new toric lens calculation calculators and toric IOLs formulas; the post operation care of toric IOLs and re-rotation of misaligned toric IOLs; and some relevant issues on multifocal toric intraocular lens. Meanwhile, this chapter also discussed toric IOL in some special cases like keratoconus corneal ectatic disorders, post-refractive surgery and post-keratoplasty, etc.

Keywords: astigmatism, cataract, toric IOL

1. Introduction

Up to more than one-third of cataract patients have preoperative corneal astigmatism of more than 1.0 diopter (D) [1], while 26.2% have more than 1.5 D [2, 3], 8–14.9% have more than 2.0 [1, 3], and 2.6–7.4% have more than 3.0 D [1, 3]. Astigmatism is one of the most important factors that affect postoperative vision quality. More than 0.5 D of residual astigmatism can reduce visual performance and patient satisfaction [4–6]. Currently, implanting a toric lens is recognized as the most accurate form of astigmatic correction during cataract surgery, especially astigmatism of more than 1 D [7]. Actually, toric IOLs correct preexisting regular corneal astigmatism usually ranging from 0.75 to 4.75 D [8]. However, the outcomes after toric IOL implantation are still influenced by many factors including accurate preoperative measurement of corneal astigmatism, IOL selection, marking techniques, intraoperative alignment and postoperative care, etc.

2. A short history and clinical outcomes of toric IOLs

The first article reporting a toric IOL (Nidek NT -98B) was published in 1994 [9], which had a cylinder power of 2.00 or 3.00 D. In the study, Shimizu et al. had relatively positive results, although some negative results still occurred in some eyes of which the lens axis rotated more than 30° [9]. Ever since then, with the predictability increasing and the safety enhancing, toric IOLs have definitely become a considerable option to correct significant astigmatism when undergoing cataract surgery [10, 11]. At present, standard toric IOLs are available in cylinder powers of 1.0 to 6.0 D, while higher cylinder powers are also available (see **Table 1**).

Toric IOL had achieved increasingly great visual outcomes. An uncorrected distance visual acuity (UDVA) of 20/40 or better is achieved in more than 70% of

IOL	Material	Design	Aspheric	Spherical power (D)	Cylinder power (D) at IOL plane	Incision size (mm)
Acri. comfort (Carl Zeiss Meditec) [12]	Hydrophilic acrylic with hydrophobic surface	Plate haptic, 11.0-mm dialect	Y	−10.0 to +32.0	1.0–12.0 (0.50 steps)	<2.0
T-flex (Rayner) [13]	Hydrophilic acrylic	C-loop haptic with AVH technology, 12.0–12.5-mm dialect	Y	−10.0 to +35.0	1.0–11.0 (0.25 steps)	<2.0
AF-1 Toric (Hoya) [7]	Hydrophobic acrylic with PMMA haptic tips	PMMA-modified C-loop haptic, 12.5-mm dialect	Y	+6.0 to +30.0	1.5–6.0 (0.75 steps)	2.0
AcrySof (Alcon) [14–19]	Hydrophobic acrylic	C-loop haptic, 13.0-mm dialect	Y	+6.0 to +34.0	1.0–6.0 (0.75 steps)	2.2
TECNIS Toric IOL (Abbott Medical Optics) [20]	Hydrophobic acrylic	"Tri-Fix" modified C haptic integral with optic, 13.0-mm dialect	Y	+5.0 to +34.0	1.5–6 (0.5–1.0 steps)	2.2
Precizon toric IOL (OPHTEC) [21, 22]	Hydrophilic acrylic	Biconvex transitional conic toric design offset-shaped haptic	Y	+1.0 to +34.0	1.0–10.0 (0.5 steps)	2.2
Morcher 89A, 92S (Morcher GmbH) [23, 24]	Hydrophilic acrylic	Bag-in-the-lens, 7.5-mm dialect	N	+10.0 to +30.0 D	0.5–8.0 (0.25 steps)	2.5
LENTIS Tplus (Oculentis) [7]	Hydrophilic acrylic with hydrophobic surface	C/Plate haptic, 12.0–11.0-mm dialect	Y	−10.0 to +35.0	0.25–12.0 (0.75–1.0 steps)	2.6
STAAR (STAAR Surgical Company) [25]	Silicone	Plate haptic, 10.8–11.2-mm dialect	N	+9.5 to +28.5	2.0 or 3.5	2.8
Light-adjustable lens (Calhoun Vision) [26]	Silicone with PMMA haptics	Modified C-loop PMMA haptics, 13.0-mm dialect	Y	+17.0 to +24.0	0.75–2.0	3.0
Microsil (HumanOptics) [27]	Silicone with PMMA haptics	C-loop haptic, 11.6-mm dialect	N	−10.0 to +35.0	1.0–15.0 (1.0 steps)	3.4

Table 1.
Summary of commercially available toric IOLs.

the cases, and spectacle independence has been reported in more than 60% of the patients in previous studies [12, 13, 15–23, 25–30], which is significantly increased compared with nontoric monofocal IOLs [31, 32]. A randomized controlled trial (RCT) compared the outcomes of AcrySof toric IOLs with conventional spherical IOLs and observed a UDVA of 20/40 or better in 92.2% of cases undergoing toric IOL implantation, with 63.4% having a UDVA of 20/25 or better. In contrast, only 81.4% of cases undergoing nontoric IOL implantation had a UDVA of 20/40 or better and 41.4% had a UDVA of 20/25 or better [9]. Similar results were found in another high-quality RCT [29].

Compared with incisional astigmatic keratotomy, toric IOLs offered better predictability and stability of correction [17], especially in moderate to high astigmatism [30]. In a recent meta-analysis (including 13 RCTs with 707 eyes), toric IOLs provided better distance visual acuity and lower amounts of residual astigmatism, combined with greater spectacle independence, than nontoric IOLs even when relaxing incisions were used [33].

From a social cost-effectiveness perspective, toric IOLs were inferior to monofocal IOLs in a recent prospective study [34], which should be noted in healthcare decision-making.

3. The measurement of astigmatism

For a toric IOL, the keratometric astigmatism (both axis and magnitude) of the cornea must be accurately measured.

3.1 Anterior corneal curvature

Traditionally, keratometry and topography take into account only the anterior corneal curvature [35]. However, nomograms predict total corneal astigmatism based on the power and axis of the anterior corneal astigmatism, assuming a fixed ratio between the anterior and posterior curvature [36]. These methods obviously cannot take outliers and irregularities into account (e.g., post-refractive surgery eyes) [35], thus leading to significant postoperative and/or overcorrection. However, if the agreement of measurement of astigmatism between instruments of different kinds is poor (more than 10°), the selection of toric IOLs requires extra care.

3.2 Posterior corneal curvature

The astigmatism of posterior cornea is generally minus lens of against-the-rule. As mentioned above, ignoring effects of actual posterior corneal curvature may lead to inaccuracies in total astigmatism estimation in some eyes. In a recent study [36], for those eyes who received IOLs with 2 diopters of cylinder or less, a coefficient of adjustment of 0.75 for with-the-rule astigmatism and 1.41 for against-the-rule astigmatism can be applied to the corneal astigmatism power value to calculate a more appropriate IOL cylinder power than that be calculated by using unadjusted anterior corneal curvature measurements.

Since minimizing the residual refractive error is especially critical in toric multifocal IOLs [37], imaging systems that measure posterior corneal curvature, as well as the new algorithm that incorporates the effect of posterior corneal astigmatism, are increasingly being invented. For example, the Scheimpflug imaging systems, slit scanning systems, and OCT systems could measure posterior corneal curvature, besides the anterior curvature. In a comparative study [35] including a Scheimpflug tomography (OCULUS Pentacam), a Placido topographer (Tomey TMS-5 in Placido mode), a swept source/Fourier domain OCT (CASIA SS-1000), an autokeratometer (Haag-Streit Lenstar), and a hybrid topographer (Tomey TMS-5), the OCULUS Pentacam has the disadvantage of high measuring noise on posterior corneal curvature. Meanwhile, the highest precision for planning toric IOL power and axis was achieved by combining the keratometry and OCT data. In a recent study, Lu et al. found that a novel multicolored spot reflection topographer system could provide high repeatable measurements in (both anterior and posterior) corneal power and astigmatism [38].

3.3 Surgically induced astigmatism

Besides naturally occurring astigmatism, the surgically induced astigmatism (SIA) is also an important factor for the appropriate option of a toric IOL. The SIA could be influenced by position and length of incisions [39]. Meanwhile, to achieve minimum residual refractive astigmatism for specific patients, the incisions could be determined by the magnitude and axis of preoperative keratometric astigmatism [4]. The application of femtosecond laser-assisted cataract surgery (FLACS) could minimize SIA.

4. IOL power calculation

An accurate biometry is a precondition not only for toric IOLs but also for regular IOL power calculation. The axial length may be measured by either ultrasonic biometry or optical systems, and SRK/T, Holladay 2, Hoffer Q, and Barrett formula are recommended to be used to calculate sphere power. Nguyen et al. adjusted the power of an existing hydrophobic acrylic IOL by a femtosecond laser [40], which is definitely a promising idea.

There are several toric calculators available for surgical planning that have been developed to predict postoperative cylinder power, such as Barrett toric calculator [41], Holladay toric calculator, and Alcon toric calculator(the revised Alcon toric calculator is a derivation of the Barrett calculator). In general, an ideal IOL power calculation formula should take into account the posterior corneal curvature, the effective lens position (ELP), as well as the SIA. And there are a few formulas available such as Abulafia-Koch linear regression formula [42], Baylor nomogram (a method from Koch) [43], Barrett formula, Abulafia-Koch formula, etc.

4.1 IOL power calculation considering posterior cornea

A few online toric IOL calculators have been revised to take into account the contribution of the posterior cornea in IOL power calculation, but it proved itself valuable. The Baylor nomogram which incorporates the posterior corneal curvature has been observed to be more precise than traditional Alcon and Holladay toric calculator without posterior corneal astigmatism compensation [44]. However, the revised AcrySof toric calculator incorporates the Barrett toric algorithm, which takes into account both the ELP and the posterior corneal astigmatism, and had better predictability than the Baylor nomogram as well as Holladay and traditional Alcon toric calculator [44]. Other toric IOL calculators such as TECNIS calculator also incorporate posterior corneal astigmatism compensation.

4.2 IOL power calculation considering ELP

Failing to consider the anterior chamber depth and cornea thickness may result in inaccurate calculations, especially in eyes with extremes of axial lengths [45]. As mentioned above, the revised AcrySof online toric calculator and iTrace toric planner takes into account the ELP [14, 46]. The TECNIS calculator incorporates the anterior chamber depth based on the axial length and keratometry values [46], and the Holladay formula incorporates the ELP in its calculations.

4.3 Intraoperative wavefront aberrometry

Intraoperative wavefront aberrometry is increasingly being used to estimate the toric IOL power and axis of placement based on the aphakic refraction, especially in post-refractive surgery cases. A recent study reported only a mean error of 0.43 ± 0.33 D with Optiwave Refractive Analysis (ORA; WaveTec Vision Systems Inc., CA, USA) in post laser-assisted in situ keratomileusis (LASIK) cases undergoing toric IOL implantation, which were more accurate than those obtained by the standard SRK/T formula and the online ASCRS calculator.

5. Surgery techniques

Many issues, such as accurate marking technique, clear corneal incisions, intraoperative alignment of the toric IOL, capsulorhexis, and IOL centration, play a significant role in achieving optimal outcomes.

5.1 Marking techniques

Preoperative reference and axis marking techniques could be broadly categorized as manual methods, image-guided systems, and intraoperative aberrometry-based methods.

The three-step manual technique is at present most commonly used [47], which is fairly accurate [48]. The first step is preoperative marking of the reference axis, which is commonly placed in the horizontal 3'o and 9'o clock positions. The second step is intraoperative alignment of the reference mark. The marking may be performed with a skin marking pen or needle. The patient should be sitting erect in a straight-ahead gaze while marking the reference axis. A change in patient position from sitting to supine may induce significant cyclotorsion; studies reported up to 28° of cyclotorsion in 68% of cases [49]. The manual marking methods have been limited by smudging of the dye, irregular, and broad marks.

Image-guided systems and intraoperative aberrometry have advantages compared with manual marking. The image-guided system based on the concept of landmarks to place the axis marks [50], which could be iris crypts, nevi, brush fields, etc. The systems capture a preoperative reference image and calculated the location of these marks and their distance in degrees from the target IOL axis. Then the system generated a final plan which provides simple angular directions from each reference mark to the planned axis of IOL placement.

There are a few image-guided systems at present such as CALLISTO Eye and Z Align (Carl Zeiss Meditec, Jena, Germany), VERION (Alcon, Fort Worth, Texas), TrueGuide (TrueVision 3D Surgical System, Santa Barbara, Calif), Osher Toric Alignment System (OTAS, Haag-Streit, Koeniz, Switzerland), and iTrace System (Tracey Technologies, Houston, Tx). Besides alignment, image-guided systems also contribute to planning the incisions, capsulorhexis size, and optimal IOL centration.

5.2 Intraoperative toric IOL alignment

Intraoperative IOL positioning is the key procedure to sustain rotation stability. During IOL alignment, the IOL should be left about 3–5° anticlockwise of the final desired lens position, followed by complete OVD removal and hydration of the wounds. Most open-loop IOLs can be rotated only clockwise, and a complete re-rotation will be needed if the IOL rotates further clockwise of the target axis.

The image-guided systems and intraoperative aberrometry could be definitely more useful than manual alignment. As mentioned above, the image-guided systems capture a preoperative reference image and an intraoperative image and then match the two images with respect to each other using landmarks. During the operation, a graphic overlay is then superimposed on the surgical field along the target axis, which provides a guide for toric IOL alignment. The image-guided systems and intraoperative aberrometry have improved the precision of toric IOL alignment, with <5° of deviation from the intended axis in the majority of cases.

Compared with manual marking, Elhofi et al. had observed more precise alignment with VERION image-guided system [51], which offers comprehensive astigmatism management, the incision location optimization, toric IOL power calculation, as well as decreasing SIA.

However, Solomon et al. claimed that, compared with the surgeon's standard of care, the use of the VERION combined with intraoperative aberrometry (Optiwave Refractive Analysis system with VerifEye) did not significantly optimize the outcomes [52]. The accuracy of CALLISTO Eye is also very effective [53], and it also assists in planning the position of limbal relaxing incisions.

6. Complications

Postoperative toric IOL misalignment is the major complication after toric IOL implantation. Toric IOL misalignment could harm visual quality. In a recent experimental study, 5° IOL axis rotation from the intended position determined a decay in the image quality of 7.03%, 10° of IOL rotation caused 11.09% decay, and 30° rotation caused 45.85% decay [54].

Toric IOL misalignment may be attributed to three factors: (1) inaccurate preoperative prediction of the axis of IOL alignment; (2) inaccurate intraoperative alignment; and (3) postoperative IOL rotation. IOL rotation may be observed as early as 1 hour after surgery, and a majority of rotations occur within the initial 10 days [18]. Early IOL rotation likely results from incomplete OVD removal, whereas late postoperative rotation is influenced by the IOL architecture, design, and axial length. In a recently published case report, the toric IOL was rotated more than 115° shortly after a neodymium: YAG (Nd:YAG) laser posterior capsulotomy [55].

Rotational stability of the IOL varies with design and material and strength of IOL capsular bag adhesions. Maximum rotational stability has been observed with hydrophobic acrylic lenses, followed by Hydrophobic acrylic, hydrophilic acrylic, PMMA and silicone. Loop haptic IOLs are better than plate-haptic IOLs on postoperative rotation stability when using silicone IOL, but they are similar when using acrylic IOL. A study of AT TORBI 709 M, which had one-piece hydrophilic acrylic with hydrophobic surface and a supporting four-haptic design, had rotation of more than 5° in 10% cases in 6 months [56]. Another study of AT TORBI 709 M reported 13% eyes had rotation of more than 10° [57], while another study reported 100% rotation of more than 10° [58]. Scialdone et al. found similar results in rotation stability between AT TORBI 709 M and AcrySof toric IOLs [59]. A long-term of 2-year study of AcrySof toric IOLs (hydrophobic acrylic IOL with Flexible loop haptic) reported postoperative rotation of more than 10° in 1.68% eyes, more than 5° in 23.3% eyes [18]. A recent cohort study [60] of 1273 eyes showed that AcrySof toric IOL was less likely to rotate, with 91.9% of eyes rotated 5° in AcrySof toric IOL eyes compared with 81.8% in TECNIS Toric IOL eyes (P < 0.0001); rotation 10° (97.8% Acrysof vs. 93.2% TECNIS, P = 0.0002) and 15° (98.6% Acrysof vs. 96.4% TECNIS, P = 0.02). Furthermore, a hydrophilic IOL with C-flex design

(Rayner 600S IOL) was reported to have excellent rotational stability: average 1.83° ± 1.44° at 6 months and no lens rotated more than 5° [61].

In cases with more than 10° of rotation, realignment of the toric IOL is needed [62]. In a study by Oshika et al., 6431 eyes are implanted with toric IOLs, and realignment was performed in 0.653% of cases [63]. An early repositioning performed after 1 week of primary cataract surgery had optical outcomes.

IOL tilt could also induce astigmatism: tilting toric IOLs aligned at 180° would decrease with-the-rule astigmatism, bringing in undercorrection, while aligned at 90° increased against-the-rule astigmatism, bringing in overcorrection [64].

Meanwhile, LASIK, customized surface ablation, or femtosecond laser-assisted intrastromal keratotomies could also be used to correct residual astigmatism [65]. Some toric rotation check, such as https://www.astigmatismfix.com/, could help determine the amount of IOL rotation, and the expected residual refraction. When the large residual cylinder not amenable to correction by rotation alone or refractive surgery, an IOL exchange, piggyback IOLs procedures may be considered.

7. Multifocal toric IOLs

Toric designs are even more required in multifocal IOLs [66] because patients undergoing multifocal IOLs may not tolerate residual astigmatism of <1 D, and multifocal IOLs without toric design perform best with less than 0.75 D of cylinder [67].

In previous studies [68–72], toric multifocal IOLs achieved good visual performance, with UDVA better than 20/40 in more than 97% of patients, uncorrected near visual acuity better than 20/40 in 100% of patients, spectacle independence in more than 80% of patients, and residual refractive astigmatism lower than 0.50 D in 38–79% of patients. Toric trifocal IOLs such as a trifocal spherical hydrophilic IOL (FineVision POD F) [73] also showed great performance.

But on the other hand, the selection of multifocal toric IOLs should be more restricted than monofocal toric IOLs, especially for the following candidates: (1) patients who had unrealistic expectations of visual quality when having related ocular comorbidities; (2) patients who may not tolerate dysphoric symptoms such as glare and halos; and (3) patients who had specific contraindications for multifocal IOLs, such as abnormal κ or α angle, etc. Thus, a comprehensive ocular examination should be undertaken to rule out any ocular comorbidities that may interfere with the postoperative outcomes.

8. Special cases

Normally, cases with irregular astigmatism, corneal ectatic disorders, post-refractive surgery, post-keratoplasty, and high myopia are not ideal candidates for toric IOL implantation, partly because they are unlikely to achieve complete refractive correction with toric IOLs. However, the amount of astigmatism may be partly reduced, decreasing spectacle dependence. And such cases may be considered for surgery after adequate counseling. As a consequence, the applications of toric IOLs are expanding to include special cases such as pellucid marginal degeneration [74, 75], mild keratoconus with cataract [76], astigmatism after keratoplasty [77–80], and high astigmatism [81]; even toric trifocal IOLs were used in high astigmatism cases [82]. In general, the indications of toric IOL are still controversial and expanding.

9. Conclusions

The outcomes after toric IOL implantation are influenced by a few factors: accurate astigmatism measurement, marking techniques, intraoperative alignment, and postoperative care. The importance of posterior corneal curvature is increasingly being recognized, and advanced toric calculators and fumulars that account for both the anterior and posterior corneal power are becoming the standard of care. The image-guided systems and intraoperative aberrometry could provide a markless IOL alignment and optimize incisions, capsulorhexis size, and optimal IOL centration. New toric IOLs with superior design are still being looked forward although they have already achieved great performance.

Acknowledgements

Thanks to my wife, Wenzhe Li, who dedicated her precious time to help when I finish this manuscript. Also, this research was supported by the Chinese Capital Clinical Features Key Project—Clinical Application on Chinese Keratoprosthesis (Project No: Z161100000516012), National Natural Science Foundation of China (Grant No. 81770887), and National Natural Science Foundation of China (Grant No. 81670830).

Conflict of interest

The authors have declared that no competing interests exist.

Other declarations

The datasets used and/or analyzed during the current study are available from the corresponding author on reasonable request.

Abbreviations

D	diopter
IOL	intraocular lens
RCT	randomized control trial
UDVA	uncorrected distance visual acuity
SIA	surgically induced astigmatism
FLACS	femtosecond laser-assisted cataract surgery
ELP	effective lens position
LASIK	laser-assisted in situ keratomileusis
ORA	Optiwave Refractive Analysis
UNVA	uncorrected near visual acuity

Author details

Zequan Xu
Department of Ophthalmology, First Medical Center, Chinese People's Liberation Army General Hospital (PLAGH), Beijing, P.R. China

*Address all correspondence to: xuzequan1986@sjtu.edu.cn

© 2019 The Author(s). Licensee IntechOpen. This chapter is distributed under the terms of the Creative Commons Attribution License (http://creativecommons.org/licenses/by/3.0), which permits unrestricted use, distribution, and reproduction in any medium, provided the original work is properly cited.

References

[1] Hoffmann PC, Hutz WW. Analysis of biometry and prevalence data for corneal astigmatism in 23,239 eyes. Journal of Cataract and Refractive Surgery. 2010;**36**(9):1479-1485. DOI: 10.1016/j.jcrs.2010.02.025

[2] Olson RJ, Braga-Mele R, Chen SH, Miller KM, Pineda R, et al. Cataract in the adult eye preferred practice pattern ((R)). Ophthalmology. 2017;**124**(2):P1-P119. DOI: 10.1016/j.ophtha.2016.09.027

[3] Mohammadi M, Naderan M, Pahlevani R, Jahanrad A. Prevalence of corneal astigmatism before cataract surgery. International Ophthalmology. 2016;**36**(6):807-817. DOI: 10.1007/s10792-016-0201-z

[4] Holladay JT, Pettit G. Improving toric intraocular lens calculations using total surgically induced astigmatism for a 2.5 mm temporal incision. Journal of Cataract and Refractive Surgery. 2019;**45**(3):272-283. DOI: 10.1016/j.jcrs.2018.09.028

[5] Villegas EA, González C, Bourdoncle B, Bonnin T, Artal P. Correlation between optical and psychophysical parameters as a function of defocus. Optometry and Vision Science. 2002;**79**(1):60-67

[6] Villegas EA, Alcón E, Artal P. Minimum amount of astigmatism that should be corrected. Journal of Cataract and Refractive Surgery. 2014;**40**(1):13-19

[7] Kaur M, Shaikh F, Falera R, Titiyal JS. Optimizing outcomes with toric intraocular lenses. Indian Journal of Ophthalmology. 2017;**65**(12):1301-1313. DOI: 10.4103/ijo.IJO_810_17

[8] Khan MI, Ch'ng SW, Muhtaseb M. The use of toric intraocular lens to correct astigmatism at the time of cataract surgery. Oman Journal of Ophthalmology. 2015;**8**(1):38

[9] Shimizu K, Misawa A, Suzuki Y. Toric intraocular lenses: Correcting astigmatism while controlling axis shift. Journal of Cataract and Refractive Surgery. 1994;**20**(5):523-526

[10] Visser N, Bauer NJ, Nuijts RM. Toric Intraocular Lenses in Cataract Surgery. London: Intech Open Access Publisher; 2012:268-292

[11] Agresta B, Knorz MC, Donatti C, Jackson D. Visual acuity improvements after implantation of toric intraocular lenses in cataract patients with astigmatism: A systematic review. BMC Ophthalmology. 2012;**12**(1):41

[12] Alio JL, Agdeppa MC, Pongo VC, El Kady B. Microincision cataract surgery with toric intraocular lens implantation for correcting moderate and high astigmatism: Pilot study. Journal of Cataract and Refractive Surgery. 2010;**36**(1):44-52. DOI: 10.1016/j.jcrs.2009.07.043

[13] Entabi M, Harman F, Lee N, Bloom PA. Injectable 1-piece hydrophilic acrylic toric intraocular lens for cataract surgery: Efficacy and stability. Journal of Cataract and Refractive Surgery. 2011;**37**(2):235-240. DOI: 10.1016/j.jcrs.2010.08.040

[14] Savini G, Hoffer KJ, Ducoli P. A new slant on toric intraocular lens power calculation. Journal of Refractive Surgery. 2013;**29**(5):348-354. DOI: 10.3928/1081597X-20130415-06

[15] Kim MH, Chung TY, Chung ES. Long-term efficacy and rotational stability of AcrySof toric intraocular lens implantation in cataract surgery. Korean Journal of Ophthalmology. 2010;**24**(4):207-212. DOI: 10.3341/kjo.2010.24.4.207

[16] Koshy JJ, Nishi Y, Hirnschall N, Crnej A, Gangwani V, et al. Rotational stability of a single-piece toric acrylic intraocular lens. Journal of Cataract and

Refractive Surgery. 2010;**36**(10): 1665-1670. DOI: 10.1016/j.jcrs.2010.05.018

[17] Titiyal JS, Agarwal T, Jhanji V. Toric intraocular lens versus opposite clear corneal incisions to correct astigmatism in eyes having cataract surgery. Journal of Cataract and Refractive Surgery. 2009;**35**(10):1834-1835. DOI: 10.1016/j.jcrs.2009.05.037

[18] Miyake T, Kamiya K, Amano R, Iida Y, Tsunehiro S, et al. Long-term clinical outcomes of toric intraocular lens implantation in cataract cases with preexisting astigmatism. Journal of Cataract and Refractive Surgery. 2014; **40**(10):1654-1660. DOI: 10.1016/j.jcrs.2014.01.044

[19] Mendicute J, Irigoyen C, Aramberri J, Ondarra A, Montes-Mico R. Foldable toric intraocular lens for astigmatism correction in cataract patients. Journal of Cataract and Refractive Surgery. 2008; **34**(4):601-607. DOI: 10.1016/j.jcrs.2007.11.033

[20] Lubinski W, Kazmierczak B, Gronkowska-Serafin J, Podboraczynska-Jodko K. Clinical outcomes after uncomplicated cataract surgery with implantation of the tecnis toric intraocular lens. Journal of Ophthalmology. 2016;**2016**:3257217. DOI: 10.1155/2016/3257217

[21] Thomas BC, Khoramnia R, Auffarth GU, Holzer MP. Clinical outcomes after implantation of a toric intraocular lens with a transitional conic toric surface. The British Journal of Ophthalmology. 2018;**102**(3): 313-316. DOI: 10.1136/bjophthalmol-2017-310386

[22] Ferreira TB, Berendschot TT, Ribeiro FJ. Clinical outcomes after cataract surgery with a new transitional toric intraocular lens. Journal of Refractive Surgery. 2016;**32**(7):452-459. DOI: 10.3928/1081597X-20160428-07

[23] Rozema JJ, Gobin L, Verbruggen K, Tassignon MJ. Changes in rotation after implantation of a bag-in-the-lens intraocular lens. Journal of Cataract and Refractive Surgery. 2009;**35**(8):1385-1388. DOI: 10.1016/j.jcrs.2009.03.037

[24] Tassignon MJ, Gobin L, Mathysen D, Van Looveren J. Clinical results after spherotoric intraocular lens implantation using the bag-in-the-lens technique. Journal of Cataract and Refractive Surgery. 2011;**37**(5):830-834. DOI: 10.1016/j.jcrs.2010.12.042

[25] Ruhswurm I, Scholz U, Zehetmayer M, Hanselmayer G, Vass C, et al. Astigmatism correction with a foldable toric intraocular lens in cataract patients. Journal of Cataract and Refractive Surgery. 2000;**26**(7):1022-1027

[26] Chayet A, Sandstedt C, Chang S, Rhee P, Tsuchiyama B, et al. Use of the light-adjustable lens to correct astigmatism after cataract surgery. The British Journal of Ophthalmology. 2010; **94**(6):690-692. DOI: 10.1136/bjo.2009.164616

[27] De Silva DJ, Ramkissoon YD, Bloom PA. Evaluation of a toric intraocular lens with a Z-haptic. Journal of Cataract and Refractive Surgery. 2006;**32**(9):1492-1498. DOI: 10.1016/j.jcrs.2006.04.022

[28] Vale C, Menezes C, Firmino-Machado J, Rodrigues P, Lume M, et al. Astigmatism management in cataract surgery with precizon® toric intraocular lens: A prospective study. Clinical Ophthalmology. 2016;**10**: 151-159. DOI: 10.2147/OPTH.S91298

[29] Holland E, Lane S, Horn JD, Ernest P, Arleo R, et al. The AcrySof Toric intraocular lens in subjects with cataracts and corneal astigmatism: A randomized, subject-masked, parallel-group, 1-year study. Ophthalmology. 2010;**117**(11):2104-2111. DOI: 10.1016/j.ophtha.2010.07.033

[30] Roberts TV, Sharwood P, Hodge C, Roberts K, Sutton G. Comparison of Toric intraocular lenses and Arcuate corneal relaxing incisions to correct moderate to high astigmatism in cataract surgery. The Asia-Pacific Journal of Ophthalmology. 2014;3(1):9-16. DOI: 10.1097/APO.0b013e3182a0af21

[31] Lane SS, Ernest P, Miller KM, Hileman KS, Harris B, et al. Comparison of clinical and patient-reported outcomes with bilateral AcrySof toric or spherical control intraocular lenses. Journal of Refractive Surgery. 2009;25(10):899-901

[32] Ruiz-Mesa R, Carrasco-Sanchez D, Diaz-Alvarez SB, Ruiz-Mateos MA, Ferrer-Blasco T, et al. Refractive lens exchange with foldable toric intraocular lens. American Journal of Ophthalmology. 2009;147(6):990-996. DOI: 10.1016/j.ajo.2009.01.004

[33] Kessel L, Andresen J, Tendal B, Erngaard D, Flesner P, et al. Toric intraocular lenses in the correction of astigmatism during cataract surgery: A systematic review and meta-analysis. Ophthalmology. 2016;123(2):275-286. DOI: 10.1016/j.ophtha.2015.10.002

[34] Simons RWP, Visser N, van den Biggelaar F, Nuijts R, Webers CAB, et al. Trial-based cost-effectiveness analysis of toric versus monofocal intraocular lenses in cataract patients with bilateral corneal astigmatism in the Netherlands. Journal of Cataract and Refractive Surgery. 2019;45(2):146-152. DOI: 10.1016/j.jcrs.2018.09.019

[35] Fabian E, Wehner W. Prediction accuracy of total keratometry compared to standard keratometry using different intraocular lens power formulas. Journal of Refractive Surgery. 2019;35(6):362-368. DOI: 10.3928/1081597X-20190422-02

[36] Goggin M, Zamora-Alejo K, Esterman A, van Zyl L. Adjustment of anterior corneal astigmatism values to incorporate the likely effect of posterior corneal curvature for toric intraocular lens calculation. Journal of Refractive Surgery. 2015;31(2):98-102. DOI: 10.3928/1081597X-20150122-04

[37] Canovas C, Alarcon A, Rosen R, Kasthurirangan S, Ma JJK, et al. New algorithm for toric intraocular lens power calculation considering the posterior corneal astigmatism. Journal of Cataract and Refractive Surgery. 2018;44(2):168-174. DOI: 10.1016/j.jcrs.2017.11.008

[38] Lu W, Miao Y, Li Y, Hu X, Hu Q, et al. Comparison of multicolored spot reflection topographer and Scheimpflug-Placido system in corneal power and astigmatism measurements with Normal and post-refractive patients. Journal of Refractive Surgery. 2019;35(6):370-376. DOI: 10.3928/1081597X-20190510-01

[39] Hayashi K, Yoshida M, Hirata A, Yoshimura K. Changes in shape and astigmatism of total, anterior, and posterior cornea after long versus short clear corneal incision cataract surgery. Journal of Cataract and Refractive Surgery. 2018;44(1):39-49. DOI: 10.1016/j.jcrs.2017.10.037

[40] Nguyen J, Werner L, Ludlow J, Aliancy J, Ha L, et al. Intraocular lens power adjustment by a femtosecond laser: In vitro evaluation of power change, modulation transfer function, light transmission, and light scattering in a blue light-filtering lens. Journal of Cataract and Refractive Surgery. 2018;44(2):226-230. DOI: 10.1016/j.jcrs.2017.09.036

[41] Gundersen KG, Potvin R. Clinical outcomes with toric intraocular lenses planned using an optical low coherence reflectometry ocular biometer with a new toric calculator. Clinical Ophthalmology. 2016;10:2141-2147. DOI: 10.2147/opth.s120414

[42] Abulafia A, Koch DD, Wang L, Hill WE, Assia EI, et al. New regression formula for toric intraocular lens calculations. Journal of Cataract and Refractive Surgery. 2016;**42**(5):663-671. DOI: 10.1016/j.jcrs.2016.02.038

[43] Koch DD, Jenkins RB, Weikert MP, Yeu E, Wang L. Correcting astigmatism with toric intraocular lenses: Effect of posterior corneal astigmatism. Journal of Cataract and Refractive Surgery. 2013;**39**(12):1803-1809. DOI: 10.1016/j.jcrs.2013.06.027

[44] Abulafia A, Barrett GD, Kleinmann G, Ofir S, Levy A, et al. Prediction of refractive outcomes with toric intraocular lens implantation. Journal of Cataract and Refractive Surgery. 2015;**41**(5):936-944

[45] Savini G, Hoffer KJ, Carbonelli M, Ducoli P, Barboni P. Influence of axial length and corneal power on the astigatic power of toric intraocular lenses. Journal of Cataract and Refractive Surgery. 2013;**39**(12): 1900-1903

[46] Park HJ, Lee H, Woo YJ, Kim EK, Seo KY, et al. Comparison of the astigmatic power of toric intraocular lenses using three Toric calculators. Yonsei Medical Journal. 2015;**56**(4): 1097-1105. DOI: 10.3349/ymj.2015.56.4.1097

[47] Ventura BV, Wang L, Weikert MP, Robinson SB, Koch DD. Surgical management of astigmatism with toric intraocular lenses. Arquivos Brasileiros de Oftalmologia. 2014;**77**(2): 125-131

[48] Visser N, Berendschot TT, Bauer NJ, Jurich J, Kersting O, et al. Accuracy of toric intraocular lens implantation in cataract and refractive surgery. Journal of Cataract and Refractive Surgery. 2011;**37**(8): 1394-1402. DOI: 10.1016/j.jcrs.2011.02.024

[49] Ciccio AE, Durrie DS, Stahl JE, Schwendeman F. Ocular cyclotorsion during customized laser ablation. Journal of Refractive Surgery. 2005; **21**(6):S772-S774

[50] Osher RH. Iris fingerprinting: New method for improving accuracy in toric lens orientation. Journal of Cataract & Refractive Surgery. 2010; **36**(2):351-352

[51] Elhofi AH, Helaly HA. Comparison between digital and manual marking for Toric intraocular lenses: A randomized trial. Medicine. 2015;**94**(38):e1618. DOI: 10.1097/md.0000000000001618

[52] Solomon KD, Sandoval HP, Potvin R. Correcting astigmatism at the time of cataract surgery: Toric IOLs and corneal relaxing incisions planned with an image-guidance system and intraoperative aberrometer versus manual planning and surgery. Journal of Cataract and Refractive Surgery. 2019;**45**(5):569-575. DOI: 10.1016/j.jcrs.2018.12.002

[53] Mayer WJ, Kreutzer T, Dirisamer M, Kern C, Kortuem K, et al. Comparison of visual outcomes, alignment accuracy, and surgical time between 2 methods of corneal marking for toric intraocular lens implantation. Journal of Cataract and Refractive Surgery. 2017;**43**(10):1281-1286. DOI: 10.1016/j.jcrs.2017.07.030

[54] Tognetto D, Perrotta AA, Bauci F, Rinaldi S, Antonuccio M, et al. Quality of images with toric intraocular lenses. Journal of Cataract & Refractive Surgery. 2018;**44**(3):376-381. DOI: 10.1016/j.jcrs.2017.10.053

[55] Kaindlstorfer C, Kneifl M, Reinelt P, Schonherr U. Rotation of a toric intraocular lens from neodymium: YAG laser posterior capsulotomy. Journal of Cataract and Refractive Surgery. 2018; **44**(4):510-511. DOI: 10.1016/j.jcrs.2018.02.018

[56] Mencucci R, Favuzza E, Guerra F, Giacomelli G, Menchini U. Clinical outcomes and rotational stability of a 4-haptic toric intraocular lens in myopic eyes. Journal of Cataract and Refractive Surgery. 2014;**40**(9):1479-1487. DOI: 10.1016/j.jcrs.2013.12.024

[57] Bascaran L, Mendicute J, Macias-Murelaga B, Arbelaitz N, Martinez-Soroa I. Efficacy and stability of AT TORBI 709 M toric IOL. Journal of Refractive Surgery. 2013;**29**(3):194-199. DOI: 10.3928/1081597x-20130129-02

[58] Kretz FT, Breyer D, Klabe K, Auffarth GU, Kaymak H. Clinical outcomes and capsular bag stability of a four-point haptic bitoric intraocular lens. Journal of Refractive Surgery. 2015;**31**(7):431-436. DOI: 10.3928/1081597x-20150518-11

[59] Scialdone A, De Gaetano F, Monaco G. Visual performance of 2 aspheric toric intraocular lenses: Comparative study. Journal of Cataract and Refractive Surgery. 2013;**39**(6):906-914. DOI: 10.1016/j.jcrs.2013.01.037

[60] Lee BS, Chang DF. Comparison of the rotational stability of two Toric intraocular lenses in 1273 consecutive eyes. Ophthalmology. 2018;**125**(9):1325-1331. DOI: 10.1016/j.ophtha.2018.02.012

[61] Bhogal-Bhamra GK, Sheppard AL, Kolli S, Wolffsohn JS. Rotational stability and centration of a new toric lens design platform using objective image analysis over 6 months. Journal of Refractive Surgery. 2019;**35**(1):48-53. DOI: 10.3928/1081597X-20181204-01

[62] Felipe A, Artigas JM, Diez-Ajenjo A, Garcia-Domene C, Alcocer P. Residual astigmatism produced by toric intraocular lens rotation. Journal of Cataract and Refractive Surgery. 2011;**37**(10):1895-1901. DOI: 10.1016/j.jcrs.2011.04.036

[63] Oshika T, Inamura M, Inoue Y, Ohashi T, Sugita T, et al. Incidence and outcomes of repositioning surgery to correct misalignment of Toric intraocular lenses. Ophthalmology. 2017;**125**(1):31-35. DOI: 10.1016/j.ophtha.2017.07.004

[64] Weikert MP, Golla A, Wang L. Astigmatism induced by intraocular lens tilt evaluated via ray tracing. Journal of Cataract & Refractive Surgery. 2018;**44**(6):745-749. DOI: 10.1016/j.jcrs.2018.04.035

[65] Ruckl T, Dexl AK, Bachernegg A, Reischl V, Riha W, et al. Femtosecond laser-assisted intrastromal arcuate keratotomy to reduce corneal astigmatism. Journal of Cataract and Refractive Surgery. 2013;**39**(4):528-538. DOI: 10.1016/j.jcrs.2012.10.043

[66] Waltz KL, Featherstone K, Tsai L, Trentacost D. Clinical outcomes of TECNIS toric intraocular lens implantation after cataract removal in patients with corneal astigmatism. Ophthalmology. 2015;**122**(1):39-47. DOI: 10.1016/j.ophtha.2014.06.027

[67] Braga-Mele R, Chang D, Dewey S, Foster G, Henderson BA, et al. Multifocal intraocular lenses: Relative indications and contraindications for implantation. Journal of Cataract and Refractive Surgery. 2014;**40**(2):313-322. DOI: 10.1016/j.jcrs.2013.12.011

[68] Venter J, Pelouskova M. Outcomes and complications of a multifocal toric intraocular lens with a surface-embedded near section. Journal of Cataract and Refractive Surgery. 2013;**39**(6):859-866. DOI: 10.1016/j.jcrs.2013.01.033

[69] Chen XF, Zhao M, Shi YH, Yang LP, Lu Y, et al. Visual outcomes and optical quality after implantation of a diffractive multifocal toric intraocular lens. Indian Journal of Ophthalmology. 2016;**64**(4):285-291. DOI: 10.4103/0301-4738.182939

[70] Bellucci R, Bauer NJC, Daya SM, Visser N, Santin G, et al. Visual acuity and refraction with a diffractive multifocal toric intraocular lens. Journal of Cataract and Refractive Surgery. 2013;39(10):1507-1518. DOI: 10.1016/j.jcrs.2013.04.036

[71] Ferreira TB, Marques EF, Rodrigues A, Montes-Mico R. Visual and optical outcomes of a diffractive multifocal toric intraocular lens. Journal of Cataract and Refractive Surgery. 2013;39(7):1029-1035. DOI: 10.1016/j.jcrs.2013.02.037

[72] Gangwani V, Hirnschall N, Findl O, Maurino V. Multifocal toric intraocular lenses versus multifocal intraocular lenses combined with peripheral corneal relaxing incisions to correct moderate astigmatism. Journal of Cataract and Refractive Surgery. 2014;40(10):1625-1632. DOI: 10.1016/j.jcrs.2014.01.037

[73] Poyales F, Garzon N. Comparison of 3-month visual outcomes of a spherical and a toric trifocal intraocular lens. Journal of Cataract and Refractive Surgery. 2019;45(2):135-145. DOI: 10.1016/j.jcrs.2018.09.025

[74] Balestrazzi A, Baiocchi S, Balestrazzi A, Cartocci G, Tosi GM, et al. Mini-incision cataract surgery and toric lens implantation for the reduction of high myopic astigmatism in patients with pellucid marginal degeneration. Eye. 2015;29(5):637-642. DOI: 10.1038/eye.2015.13

[75] Luck J. Customized ultra-high-power toric intraocular lens implantation for pellucid marginal degeneration and cataract. Journal of Cataract and Refractive Surgery. 2010;36(7):1235-1238. DOI: 10.1016/j.jcrs.2010.04.009

[76] Kamiya K, Shimizu K, Miyake T. Changes in astigmatism and corneal higher-order aberrations after phacoemulsification with toric intraocular lens implantation for mild keratoconus with cataract. Japanese Journal of Ophthalmology. 2016;60(4):302-308. DOI: 10.1007/s10384-016-0449-x

[77] Lockington D, Wang EF, Patel DV, Moore SP, McGhee CN. Effectiveness of cataract phacoemulsification with toric intraocular lenses in addressing astigmatism after keratoplasty. Journal of Cataract and Refractive Surgery. 2014;40(12):2044-2049. DOI: 10.1016/j.jcrs.2014.03.025

[78] Stewart CM, McAlister JC. Comparison of grafted and non-grafted patients with corneal astigmatism undergoing cataract extraction with a toric intraocular lens implant. Clinical & Experimental Ophthalmology. 2010;38(8):747-757. DOI: 10.1111/j.1442-9071.2010.02336.x

[79] Wade M, Steinert RF, Garg S, Farid M, Gaster R. Results of toric intraocular lenses for post-penetrating keratoplasty astigmatism. Ophthalmology. 2014;121(3):771-777. DOI: 10.1016/j.ophtha.2013.10.011

[80] Allard K, Zetterberg M. Toric IOL implantation in a patient with keratoconus and previous penetrating keratoplasty: A case report and review of literature. BMC Ophthalmology. 2018;18(1):215. DOI: 10.1186/s12886-018-0895-y

[81] Kersey JP, O'Donnell A, Illingworth CD. Cataract surgery with toric intraocular lenses can optimize uncorrected postoperative visual acuity in patients with marked corneal astigmatism. Cornea. 2007;26(2):133-135. DOI: 10.1097/ICO.0b013e31802be5cc

[82] Steinwender G, Schwarz L, Bohm M, Slavik-Lencova A, Hemkeppler E, et al. Visual results after implantation of a trifocal intraocular lens in high myopes. Journal of Cataract and Refractive Surgery. 2018;44(6):680-685. DOI: 10.1016/j.jcrs.2018.04.037

Section 3

Entoptic Phenomenon of Intraocular Lens

Chapter 5

Pseudophakic Dysphotopsia

Emely Zoraida Karam Aguilar

Abstract

Pseudophakic dysphotopsia is an unwanted entoptic phenomenon caused by intraocular lenses. Dysphotopsias have been classified as positive (brightness, streaks, haze, or glare) and negative (temporal arc or half-moon crescent) in the visual field. These visual phenomena seem to be well tolerated cause in the case of positive dysphotopsia, but not as well in the negative cases that sometimes discomfort to the patient. The incidence of dysphotopsia ranges from 20% to 77.7%, and the prevalence seems not to be altered by the type of intraocular lens. Pseudophakic dysphotopsia continues to be enigmatic over time; however, many efforts are being made in order to resolve the mystery. In this chapter, the evolution of the dysphotopsia, possible causes, and proposed treatments will be described.

Keywords: pseudophakic dysphotopsia, negative dysphotopsia, positive dysphotopsia, dysphotopsia, half-moon crescent

1. Introduction

Cataract surgery has been one of the great ophthalmological contributions to the worldwide prevention and treatment of blindness.

The first cataract surgery was performed by an Indian surgeon, Sushruta, in the fifth century BC. [1–3]. Over time, improvements in cataract surgery led to many advances, such as the replacement of the opaque crystalline lens with an intraocular lens (IOL). The first IOL implant was performed by Sir Harold Ridley on November 29, 1949, at St. Thomas Hospital, London [4, 5]. Thanks to the contributions of many scientists and surgeons, techniques improved as well as IOL design. However, with the use of new technologies, complications or unwanted side effects may also arise. Dysphotopsia secondary to IOL [6, 7], is the reason for this chapter.

2. Pseudophakic dysphotopsia

Dysphotopsias are visual phenomena caused by light in phakic and pseudophakic patients. The term was introduced by Tester et al. [6] in the year 2000, and included all entoptic phenomena triggered by light (glare, halos, and dark arc). These phenomena frequently bother the patient, producing a certain degree of dissatisfaction, even in circumstances where there is good visual acuity (20/20 or better).

Dysphotopsia in phakic patients may improve with correction of the refractive error [8], special lenses [9], sunglasses [10], lenses with filters [11] and other techniques. In patients with significant cataracts, surgery is the option [6].

Before the advent of IOLs, aphakic patients (without IOL) who were placed in contact lenses reported glare phenomena [11]. The first report was by Koetting and Von Gunten in 1969 [12]. Subsequently, with the emergence of IOLs, patients with pseudophakia began to experience visual phenomena more emphatically than they did before surgery [13]. However, the benefit of improvement in visual acuity generally compensated for problems with dysphotopsia. A number of clinicians and researchers have tried to determine the causes of dysphotopsia [13].

Initial reports considered causes including the pupil, the intraocular lens, and the posterior capsule. This is reflected in one of the initial publications by Doden in 1984 [14]. This author studied the pupillary changes observed in 2500 eyes operated on cataract by extra capsular technique and phacoemulsification. He associated glare with the optical irregularity caused by the pseudophakia "per-se" or the opacities affecting the posterior capsule. Subsequently, sophisticated techniques were employed, refining the studies and reducing the number of causative factors to IOL as well as opacity of the posterior capsule [1, 12, 13, 15].

Between 1994 and 1995, the 6 mm and 5.5 mm acrylic IOL were introduced, which allowed patients to have calm eyes in the postoperative period, that is, with less chance of developing anterior uveitis and cystoid macular edema. They also found that these lenses caused less fibrosis and opacities of the posterior capsule, with lower capsular contraction, reduction of optical precipitates, and good optical centering [16]. Based on this, it was postulated that the square edge of the intraocular lens was the primary reason for the above findings [15, 17, 18]. In the laboratory, Nishi [15] confirmed that the edge of the IOL acted as a barrier to cell migration within the posterior capsule independent of the material. Unfortunately, the edge also caused a new undesirable visual phenomenon resulting from internal reflection due to the angle of incidence of oblique light. This was often referred to by the patient as a dark shadow in a half moon shape or an arc in the temporal field. The effect was more annoying than previously reported, proving even difficult to predict which patient could develop this symptomatology [15, 17, 19, 20].

Pseudophakic dysphotopsia was presented for the first time by Olson, MD, at the XVIth Congress of the European Society of Cataract & Refractive Surgeons, in Nice, France, on September 1998 [7]. Initially, it was thought that this visual phenomenon was transitory. Overtime the visual effect persisted as a souce of visual compliants, resulting in a number of procedures to attempt to reduce or solve the problem. In 2000, Davidson [7] divided these dysphotopsia phenomena according to the symptoms into positive and negative.

3. Dysphotopsia classification

3.1 Positive dysphotopsia

Positive dysphotopsia refers to the brilliant, lines or = stripes that emanate from a central point of a light source sometimes creating diffusion and strong glare, described by the author as "hazy glare."

Few reports exist regarding positive dysphotopsia. Shambhu et al. [11] used a questionnaire to compare three different types of acrylic IOLs. In this study, 15 patients with severe dysphotopsia (negative and positive) were reported, but apparently, positive dysphotopsia (particularly the glare phenomena) was not severe enough to require the change of IOL. In a study conducted by Radford et al. [21], follow-up of 61 patients with Akreos Adapt and SN60-AT intraocular lenses found that dysphotopsia declined by 8 weeks in 31.3% for positive dysphotopsia and 20.7% for negative ones.

Recently, publications showed in vitro evaluations that IOL designs with round optic edge curvature and full functional optics demonstrated the lowest level of glare-type photic phenomena. Clinical studies are necessary to demonstrate this observation [22].

My personal opinion is that positive dysphotopsia is caused by the wavelength of light as it interacts with the pseudophakic lens. Intraocular lens still permits significant transmission between 350 and 400 nm. Most intraocular lenses provide a reasonable imitation of the spectral characteristics of the natural lens, but probably, the exact balance to the natural lens has not been achieved [23, 24].

In relation to the type of dysphotopsia, it seems that positive dysphotopsias are better tolerated than negative ones; the reason is for this unknown. That's why conservative treatment or observation is generally recommended. However, some authors recommend correcting the refractive error with conventional or contact lenses, while also treating coexisting ocular pathology such as the opacity of the posterior capsule requiring it, and intraocular lens decentralization or large pupil size [25].

Chandramani A et al. relate positive dysphotopsia with the square edge of IOL. The authors reported that a patient with previous refractive surgery and persistent positive dysphotopsia after the insertion of a square-edge IOL responded well when they inserted a zero-power 3-piece silicone IOL in the sulcus, in order to maintain the refractive efficacy of the original IOL. It was thought that the symptoms decreased because the rounded edge of the silicone optic masked the aberrant reflections and refractions of the square edge of the acrylic IOL [25].

3.2 Negative dysphotopsia

Negative dysphotopsia is characterized by an arc-shaped shadow, usually located in the temporal field. Visible with or without frame lenses, the problem can be monocular or binocular and may affect near and far vision as well as occur in internal or external environments (lighting or gloom), mobile or not. Negative dysphotopsia generally appears 1-2 days postoperatively. Over time, some of them disappear and in others remain.

Various approaches to negative dysphotopsia were made in search for possible solutions [7, 13, 19, 20, 26–33] as reflected below:

1. Related to the intraocular lens:

   - Anterior and posterior lens surface

     ○ Reflections associated with the anterior and posterior surface of the lens due to the high refractive index of the lens material

     ○ Reflections generated by the high index of the bright optical edge material

   - Intraocular lens edge

     ○ Straight or round

   - Reflections generated by the high index of the bright and straight optical edge material

- Diameter

- Number of lens parts

    ○ One to three pieces

2. Manufacturing:

    - Optical defect during the manufacturing process

    - Central optical defect during the folding process

3. Surgeon:

    - Incomplete capsulorhexis with optical overlap

    - Reflection of the capsulotomy of the anterior border projected into the nasal peripheral retina

    - Temporal clear corneal incision

4. Patient: visual system or psychological factors:

    - Complex interaction of a predisposed and vulnerable pseudophakic visual system

    - Dark irises

    - Prominent eyeballs

    - Deep orbits

    - Post negative image phenomenon

    - Neural adaptation

A program with a three-dimensional model eye was used to study the edges (straight or truncated and/or round) of IOL, through an analysis of ray tracing emanating from the light. The rays that reach the straight edge cause reflection of the light at an angle greater than 30 to 40–90° or more, maximizing the intensity of the reflexes, since they reach very close to each other and reflect on the opposite side of the peripheral retina as a dark shadow described by the patients as an arch or crescent (negative dysphotopsia). At the round edges, the rays cause significant dispersion and are reflected before 30°, not causing this temporary penumbra [7, 19, 20, 33].

It was shown that the round edge decreased the image in the form of an arc (negative dysphotopsia) by 87–91% in relation to the square edge [19]. Additional evidence of absence of positive dysphotopsia phenomena (light flashes) but not negative when the edges were compared with opaque lens was also found. Lenses with textured or opaque edges as a replacement or as a primary lens in the second eye suppose a decrease in the occurrence of positive and negative dysphotopsias. This type of design (textured or opaque border) creates the same type of light scattering as the nasal periphery of the translucent capsule, reduces the internal diffusion of light from the straight edge by scattering, but still allows the presence of positive dysphotopsia and does not make the negative ones disappear [16, 30, 34].

The opaque edges of the AcrySof SA30 IOL were compared with the bright edges in the AcrySof MA30 BA (Alcon) and AcrySof MA60BM (Alcon) intraocular lens models [7], but the negative dysphotopsia did not disappear.

The diameter of the IOL does not significantly reduce the occurrence of dysphotopsia as Davidson reported when two types of lens diameters of 5.5 and 3.60 mm were compared; the occurrence of negative dysphotopsia was similar (80%) in both groups [7].

In relation with the lens material, Tester et al. compared two types of acrylic intraocular lenses of different diameters (5.5 and 6 mm) with a control group (no acrylic IOL); the authors found that acrylic lenses produce more dysphotopsia than nonacrylic IOL. The authors concluded that patients who received an acrylic IOL with flattened edges were at increased risk of experiencing images associated with edge reflections [6]. Holladay et al. found that only the square-edged design concentrated the light into a well-formed arc on the retina. Round-edge designs tended to disperse the stray light over a much larger portion of the retina, suggesting that its visual consequences fall below a perceptible threshold [13, 19].

Radford et al. compared two types of acrylic IOL (AcrySof SN60-AT IOL (Alcon) and the Akreos Adapt (Bausch & Lomb) IOL. The results of this study showed that patients with SN60-AT IOL reported more undesired images than patients with the Akreos Adapt IOL. It was more significant during the first week postsurgery, but at 8 weeks, the incidence of this negative dysphotopsia decreased in 20.7%; the cause of this phenomenon was not clarified by the authors [21].

The anterior surface of the AcrySof MA30 BA and AcrySof MA60 BA lenses with a 5.5 D curve was studied; the remaining power was found on the posterior surface. Because these surfaces are highly reflective, it could make lenticular reflections complex enough to cause negative dysphotopsia. The optical inversion or reversion of the anterior-posterior diopter surface (posterior surface flatter than the previous one) as observed in the AcrySof MA30 AA and AcrySof SA30 AL lenses did not solve the problem [7].

The incision in the temporal area of clear cornea has been implicated by Osher [35] as a cause of transient negative dysphotopsia due to a broad clear base and incisional edema in the cornea that interferes with the oblique light projected into the distant peripheral field; however, it does not explain permanent dysphotopsia. Nasal, upper, and lower incisions and scleral tunnel showed no difference between the presence of transient and permanent negative dysphotopsia [36].

One-piece lenses in a posterior chamber with horizontally placed haptics make the edge of the lens more peripheral when the "shoulder" of the haptic is inserted into the optics; this would imply that the "shadow" would move more previously, reflecting with less amplitude, but this proposal would have to be supported by the ray tracing program [29, 37, 38].

A manufacturing defect should be evident in other intraocular lenses of the same batch used in patients, but this did not occur [7].

The central optics could be altered by folding; when folding forceps are used, an irregular line is formed temporarily, since it disappears after the operation. However, if it persists permanently, it can create defects, but they do not specifically produce negative dysphotopsia. Nowadays, with the injectors used for lens folding, no alterations have been demonstrated, even when they have been studied due to intraocular lens change [7]. Incomplete capsulorhexis with its superimposition variable is quite common; this would not explain a temporary defect of the visual field [29, 34].

Individual predisposition with a certain constellation of factors in relation to ocular anatomy, including corneal curvature, new pseudophakic state, anterior chamber depth, axial length, and intraocular lens power, can be particularly vulnerable, also be sensitive to aberration, and produce dysphotopsia. This peculiar interaction seems to vary from patient to patient [16, 33, 38].

Of all these studies, the design of the intraocular lens, specifically the edge, proved to be the source of negative pseudophakic dysphotopsia. The explanation of this enigmatic phenomenon has not been elucidated despite so many investigations [7, 34, 38].

In 2014, the author reported that the negative dysphotopsia was caused by a stimulation of the unpaired temporary crescent or "half moon" because the incidence of rays on the edge of the intraocular lenses refracts on the peripheral nasal retina outside 30° (location area of the temporary flood). The fact that some patients have it at 30° and others between 60 and 90° would explain why some patients may present them and others not, as well as unilateral or bilateral [39].

The disappearance or transientness of the negative dysphotopsia was explained by the opacification or translucency of the nasal sector of the capsule, later acting as a diffuser of the rays, in the first week or months following the surgery. The opacity of the posterior capsule causes diffusion of light and reduces contrast and retinal sensitivity. The anterior axial movement of the intraocular lens by contraction of the capsular bag maybe is another explanation that decreases the occurrence over time, since it reduces the axial space under the iris to 0.06 mm or less, causing a myopic change that is extremely rare. However, this has not made dysphotopsia disappear [38].

In relation to a persistent visual phenomenon, possible therapeutics arise such as the use of miotics [6, 21, 23, 29] but, contrary to expectations, it increases the problem and the pharmacological dilation seems to reduce it [34], anterior and posterior capsulotomies [6, 24, 34, 39, 40], smaller capsulorhexis [6, 31, 37], modifications of the intraocular lens [11, 30, 32, 34], change of intraocular lens [6, 13, 37, 40] do not solve the problem. The placement of another intraocular lens on the primary or "piggy bag" [29, 38] and reverse optical capture of the lens [34, 38] had partial or complete resolution of symptoms. The suture of the IOL-capsule complex iris bag [38] can decrease the visual phenomenon. The author used prism in the eye of dysphotopsia causing a displacement of the temporal crescent outside the visual field, with the disappearance of symptoms [39].

Henderson et al. [40] reported a 2.3-fold decrease in negative dysphotopsia symptoms early after cataract surgery when the nasal optic–haptic junction was oriented slightly super nasally (30° from horizontal) when compared with the haptic junction being oriented vertically. Henderson hypothesized that when the haptic junction was placed vertically, it exposed the nasal optic edge to reflections from temporal light. By placing the haptic junction relatively horizontal, the junction would then "block the light," and the intraocular lens edge reflections and the resultant temporal negative dysphotopsia shadow would be avoided.

Erie et al. [41] with a ray-tracing software demonstrated how the horizontal haptic junction minimizes negative dysphotopsia.

The incidence of dysphotopsia phenomena in pseudophakic patients after uncomplicated cataract surgery varies, ranging from 20 to 77.7%, since there are only isolated reports as can be seen in the literature [6, 11, 30, 39, 42–49]; however, the prevalence does not seem to be altered with the type of intraocular lens [28].

4. Conclusions

Pseudophakic dysphotopsia is an entoptic phenomenon induced by intraocular lenses that cause discomfort to patients. Positive dysphotopsia manifested as glare is well tolerated by patients, and negative dysphotopsia reported from the incorporation of intraocular lenses with square edges is a source of dissatisfaction in pseudophakia patients despite good visual acuity. After evaluating the different factors that could be responsible for it from the intraocular lens, manufacturing, surgical technique, surgeon, and patient, it was concluded that the square edge of the intraocular lens is responsible for the undesirable phenomenon. Multiple therapeutics have been proposed in order to solve the problem such as the use of miotic drops, piggy back, intraocular lens replacement textured or freezing lenses, etc. without finding the appropriate therapy. Additional studies with software or intraocular lens design program on schematic eye will be necessary to solve the problem.

Conflict of interest

The author declares no conflict of interest.

Author details

Emely Zoraida Karam Aguilar[1,2]

1 Centro Médico Docente La Trinidad, Caracas, Venezuela

2 Fundación Visión, Asunción, Paraguay

*Address all correspondence to: emelykaram@gmail.com

IntechOpen

© 2019 The Author(s). Licensee IntechOpen. This chapter is distributed under the terms of the Creative Commons Attribution License (http://creativecommons.org/licenses/by/3.0), which permits unrestricted use, distribution, and reproduction in any medium, provided the original work is properly cited.

References

[1] Raju VK. Susruta of ancient India. Indian Journal of Ophthalmology. 2003;**51**(2):119-122

[2] Roy PN, Mehra KS, Deshpande PJ. Cataract surgery performed before 800B.C. The British Journal of Ophthalmology. 1975;**59**(3):171. DOI: 10.1136/bjo.59.3.171

[3] Kansupada KB, Sassani JW. Sushruta: The father of Indian surgery and ophthalmology. Documenta Ophthalmologica. 1997;**93**(1-2):159-167

[4] Obuchowska I, Mariak Z. Sir Harold Ridley--the creator of modern cataract surgery. Klinika Oczna. 2005;**107**(4-6):382-384

[5] Kohnen T. How far we have come: From Ridley's first intraocular lens to modern IOL technology. Journal of Cataract and Refractive Surgery. 2009;**35**(12):2039. DOI: 10.1016/j.jcrs.2009.10.019

[6] Tester R, Pace NL, Samore M, Olson RJ. Dysphotopsia in phakic and pseudophakic patients: Incidence and relation to intraocular lens type (2). Journal of Cataract and Refractive Surgery. 2000;**26**(6):810-816

[7] Davison JA. Positive and negative dysphotopsia in patients with acrylic intraocular lenses. Journal of Cataract and Refractive Surgery. 2000;**26**(9):1346-1355

[8] Kwok LS, Daszynski DC, Kuznetsov VA, Pham T, Ho A, Coroneo MT. Peripheral light focusing as a potential mechanism for phakic dysphotopsia and lens phototoxicity. Ophthalmic & Physiological Optics. 2004;**24**(2):119-120

[9] Sakamoto Y, Sasaki K, Kojima M, Sasaki H, Sakamoto A, Sakai M, et al. The effects of protective eyewear on glare and crystalline lens transparency. Developments in Ophthalmology. 2002;**35**:93-103

[10] Steen R, Whitaker D, Elliott DB, Wild JM. Effect of filters on disability glare. Ophthalmic & Physiological Optics. 1993;**13**(4):371-376

[11] Shambhu S, Shanmuganathan VA, Charles SJ. The effect of lens design on dysphotopsia in different acrylic IOLs. Eye (London, England). 2005;**19**(5):567-570. DOI: 10.1038/sj.eye.6701568

[12] Koetting RA, Von Gunten TL. Glare-flare with contact lenses in aphakia. American Journal of Optometry and Archives of American Academy of Optometry. 1969;**46**(10):730-734

[13] Schwiegerling J. Recent developments in pseudophakic dysphotopsia. Current Opinion in Ophthalmology. 2006;**17**:27-30. DOI: 10.1097/01.icu.0000193065.09499.7e

[14] Doden W. Pseudophakia and the pupil. Klinische Monatsblätter für Augenheilkunde. 1984;**185**(3):155-157. DOI: 10.1055/s-2008-1054590

[15] Nishi O, Nishi K. Preventive effect of a second-generation silicone intraocular lens on posterior capsule opacification. Journal of Cataract and Refractive Surgery. 2002;**28**:1236-1240

[16] Davidson JA. Clinical performance of Alcon SA30AL and SA60AT single-piece acrylic intraocular lenses. Journal of Cataract and Refractive Surgery. 2002;**28**:1112-1123

[17] Vargas LG, Peng Q, Apple DJ, Escobar-Gomez M, Pandey SK, Arthur SN, et al. Evaluation of 3 modern single-piece foldable intraocular lenses. Clinicopathological study of posterior capsule opacification in a rabbit model. Journal of Cataract and Refractive Surgery. 2002;**28**:1241-1250

[18] Olson RJ, Mamalis N, Werner L, Apple DJ. Cataract Treatment in the Beginning of the 21st Century. American Journal of Ophthalmology. 2003;**136**:146-154. DOI: 10.1016/s0002-9394(03)00226-5

[19] Holladay JT, Lang A, Portney V. Analysis of edge glare phenomena in intraocular lens edge designs. Journal of Cataract and Refractive Surgery. 1999;**25**:748-752

[20] Coroneo MT, Pham T, Kwok LS. Off-axis edge glare in pseudophakic dysphotopsia. Journal of Cataract and Refractive Surgery. 2003;**29**(10):1969-1973

[21] Radford SW, Carlsson AM, Barrett GD. Comparison of pseudophakic dysphotopsia with Akreos Adapt and SN60-AT intraocular lenses. Journal of Cataract and Refractive Surgery. 2007;**33**(1):88-93. DOI: 10.1016/j.jcrs.2006.09.014

[22] Das KK, Werner L, Collins S, Hong X. In vitro and schematic model eye assessment of glare or positive dysphotopsia-type photic phenomena: Comparison of a new material IOL to other monofocal IOLs. Journal of Cataract and Refractive Surgery. 2019;**45**(2):219-227. DOI: 10.1016/j.jcrs.2018.09.017

[23] van Norren D, van de Kraats J. Spectral transmission of intraocular. lenses expressed as a virtual age. The British Journal of Ophthalmology. 2007;**91**(10):1374-1375. DOI: 10.1136/bjo.2007.117903

[24] Edwards KH, Gibson GA. Intraocular lens short wavelength light filtering. Clinical & Experimental Optometry. 2010;**93**(6):390-399. DOI: 10.1111/j.1444-0938.2010.00538.x

[25] Chandramani A, Riaz KM. Management of positive dysphotopsia in a patient with prior refractive surgery. Canadian Journal of Ophthalmology. 2018;**53**(1):e27-e29. DOI: 10.1016/j.jcjo.2017.06.007

[26] Marques FF, Marques DM. Unilateral dysphotopsia after bilateral intraocular lens implantation using the AR40e IOL model: Case report. Arquivos Brasileiros de Oftalmologia. 2007;**70**(2):350-354

[27] Ernest PH. Severe photic phenomenon. Journal of Cataract and Refractive Surgery. 2006;**32**(4):685-686. DOI: 10.1016/j.jcrs.2006.01.024

[28] Allen R, Ho-Yen GO, Beckingsale AB, Fitzke FW, Sciscio AG, Saleh GM. Post-capsulotomy dysphotopsia in monofocal versus multifocal lenses. Clinical & Experimental Optometry. 2009;**92**(2):104-109. DOI: 10.1111/j.1444-0938.2008.00345.x

[29] Birchall W, Brahma AK. Eccentric capsulorhexis and postoperative dysphotopsia following phacoemulsification. Journal of Cataract and Refractive Surgery. 2004;**30**(6):1378-1381. DOI: 10.1016/j.jcrs.2003.11.029

[30] Meacock WR, Spalton DJ, Khan S. The effect of texturing the intraocular lens edge on postoperative glare symptoms: A randomized, prospective, double-masked study. Archives of Ophthalmology. 2002;**120**(10):1294-1298. DOI: 10.1001/archopht.120.10.1294

[31] Wallin TR, Hincley M, Nilson C, Olson RJ. A Clinical Comparison of Single-piece and Three-piece Truncated Hydrophobic Acrylic Intraocular Lenses. American Journal of Ophthalmology. 2003;**136**:614-619. DOI: 10.1016/s0002-9394 (03)00418-5

[32] Aslam TM, Dhillon B. Effect on glare of texturing the truncated edge of an intraocular lens. Archives of

Ophthalmology. 2003;**121**(9):1345. DOI: 10.1001/archopht.121.9.1345-a

[33] Trattler WB, Whitsett JC, Simone PA. Negative dysphotopsia after intraocular lens implantation irrespective of design and material. Journal of Cataract and Refractive Surgery. 2005;**31**:841-845. DOI: 10.1016/j.jcrs.2004.12.044

[34] Masket S, Fram NR. Pseudophakic negative dysphotopsia: Surgical management and new theory of etiology. Journal of Cataract and Refractive Surgery. 2011;**37**(7):1199-1207. DOI: 10.1016/j.jcrs.2011.02.022

[35] Osher RH. Negative dysphotopsia: Long-term study and possible explanation for transient symptoms. Journal of Cataract and Refractive Surgery. 2008;**34**:1699-1707. DOI: 10.1016/j.jcrs.2008.06.026

[36] Cooke DL. Negative dysphotopsia after temporal corneal incisions. Journal of Cataract and Refractive Surgery. 2010;**36**:671-672. DOI: 10.1016/j.jcrs.2010.01.004

[37] Izak AM, Werner L, Pandey SK, Apple DJ, Vargas LG, Davison JA. Single-piece hydrophobic acrylic intraocular lens explanted within the capsular bag: Case report with clinicopathological correlation. Journal of Cataract & Refractive Surgery. 2004;**30**(6):1356-1361. DOI: 10.1016/j.jcrs.2003.09.061

[38] Holladay JT, Zhao H, Reisin CR. Negative dysphotopsia: The enigmatic penumbra. Journal of Cataract and Refractive Surgery. 2012;**38**(7):1251-1265. DOI: 10.1016/j.jcrs.2012.01.032

[39] Karam EZ. Disfotopsia pseudofáquica negativa. Fenomeno visual no deseado ocasionado por lente intraocular. Gaceta Médica de Caracas. 2014;**122**(2):121-135

[40] Henderson BA, Yi DH, Constantine JB, Geneva II. New preventative approach for negative dysphotopsia. Journal of Cataract and Refractive Surgery. 2016;**42**:1449-1455. DOI: 10.1016/j.jcrs.2016.08.020

[41] Erie JC, Simpson MJ, Bandhauer MH. Influence of the intraocular lens optic-haptic junction on illumination of the peripheral retina and negative dysphotopsia. Journal of Cataract and Refractive Surgery. 2019: 1-4. DOI: 10.1016/j.jcrs.2019.04.019

[42] Cooke DL, Kasko S, Platt LO. Resolution of negative dysphotopsia after laser anterior capsulotomy. Journal of Cataract and Refractive Surgery. 2013;**39**(7):1107-1109. DOI: 10.1016/j.jcrs.2013.05.002

[43] Folden DV. Neodymium:YAG laser anterior capsulectomy: Surgical option in the management of negative dysphotopsia. Journal of Cataract and Refractive Surgery. 2013;**39**(7):1110-1115. DOI: 10.1016/j.jcrs.2013.04.015

[44] Nadler DJ, Jaffe NS, Clayman HM, Jaffe MS, Luscombe SM. Glare disability in eyes with intraocular lenses. American Journal of Ophthalmology. 1984;**97**(1):43-47. DOI: 10.1016/0002-9394(84)90444-6

[45] Muñoz G, Albarrán-Diego C, Ferrer-Blasco T, Sakla HF, García-Lázaro S. Visual function after bilateral implantation of a new zonal refractive aspheric multifocal intraocular lens. Journal of Cataract and Refractive Surgery. 2011;**37**(11):2043-2052. DOI: 10.1016/j.jcrs.2011.05.045

[46] Chiam PJ, Chan JH, Aggarwal RK, Kasaby S. RESTOR intraocular lens implantation in cataract surgery: Quality of vision. Journal of Cataract and Refractive Surgery. 2006;**32**(9):1459-1463. DOI: 10.1016/j.jcrs.2006.04.015

[47] Kohnen T, Allen D, Boureau C, Dublineau P, Hartmann C, Mehdorn E, et al. European multicenter study of the AcrySof ReSTOR apodized diffractive intraocular lens. Ophthalmology. 2006;**113**(4):578-584. DOI: 10.1016/j.ophtha.2005.11.020

[48] Mayer S, Böhm T, Häberle H, Pham DT, Wirbelauer C. Combined implantation of monofocal and multifocal intraocular lenses for presbyopia correction in cataract patients. Klinische Monatsblätter für Augenheilkunde. 2008;**225**(9):812-817. DOI: 10.1055/s-2008-1027604

[49] Visser N, Nuijts RM, de Vries NE, Bauer NJ. Visual outcomes and patient satisfaction after cataract surgery with toric multifocal intraocular lens implantation. Journal of Cataract and Refractive Surgery. 2011;**37**(11):2034-2042. DOI: 10.1016/j.jcrs.2011.05.041

Section 4

Myopia and Phakic Intraocular Lens

Chapter 6

Pathologic Myopia: Complications and Visual Rehabilitation

*Enzo Maria Vingolo, Giuseppe Napolitano
and Lorenzo Casillo*

Abstract

High myopia, defined as refractive error of at least −6.00D or an axial length of 26.5 mm or more, can induce many modifications in eye's anatomy that can lead to complications. When high myopia is able to decrease best corrected visual acuity (BCVA) due to its complications, it is called pathologic myopia. Pathologic myopia is one of the major causes of blindness, and it represents a serious issue, since incidence of myopia and high myopia is constantly rising. For educational purposes, in this chapter, complications of pathologic myopia will be divided into anterior (when structures external to the globe or anterior to the ora serrata are involved, such as motility disturbances and cataract) and posterior (when structures posterior to the ora serrata are involved, such as lacquer cracks, chorioretinal atrophy, Fuchs maculopathy, myopic choroidal neovascularization, and retinal detachment). Many treatments are available for pathologic myopia complications depending on their type, such as vascular endothelial growth factor (anti-VEGF) injections and surgery. We will focus on visual rehabilitation interventions, such as visual biofeedback and visual aids that in many cases are the only chance that the ophthalmologist has in order to help patients suffering from pathologic myopia to use at their maximum their residual vision.

Keywords: visual rehabilitation, low-vision aids, microperimetry, high myopia, pathologic myopia complications

1. Introduction

Many modifications in normal eye anatomy and structure occur in high myopic patients. Sclera is the most external layer of the eye. In normal nonelongated eyes, scleral thickness decreases from the limbus to the equator, then increasing again to the posterior part of the eye. Normal sclera has also well-known tensile and elastic properties. In highly myopic eyes, these properties are altered with tensile strength reduced and augmented elasticity especially at the posterior pole of the globe. The reason can be searched in the alteration of its ultrastructure (which is more layered and lamellar compared to the normal sclera), in thinning and decreased diameter of the collagen fibers, and also in configuration and conformation of the collagen fibrils. In highly myopic eyes, also a remodeling of the extracellular matrix is observed during the extension of the eyeball, even if its mechanisms are not fully understood. These modifications lead to the fact that in highly myopic eyes, sclera is thinner in the part that goes posterior to the equator, while the anterior part does not show any significative difference with normal eyes. This kind of modification can contribute to the development of many complications that will be discussed in this chapter. Corneal modifications in high myopic patients are still under debate; some studies reported modifications in corneal biomechanical properties in high myopic patients, such as lower hysteresis. According to some studies [1], highly myopic patients had flatter curvature, modifications in corneal thickness, and decreased endothelial density, while other studies did not report any statistical difference in central corneal thickness (CCT) in various ranges of myopia [2]. Choroid's thickness is significantly reduced in highly elongated eyes; its thickness in foveal and parafoveal portions showed to be inversely proportional to parameters such as patient's age, myopic sferic equivalent, and axial length of the globe, with this last parameter showing to be the most consistently related. Also, distribution of choroidal thickness is altered in these eyes, with temporal and superior regions far from the fovea that show to be thicker than foveal region. Another strong predictor for choroidal thinning in high myopic patients is the presence of a posterior scleral staphyloma [3]. Furthermore, this thinning in choroidal tissue has a negative impact on retinal trophism. With regard to choroidal flow in highly myopic eyes, studies are controversial; for some of them, blood flow in choriocapillaris is augmented, while for others not. It is possible to find differences between high myopic patients and emmetropic ones even in retinal blood flow. Density of the superficial and deep plexus is significatively reduced in high myopic subjects, and the magnitude of this phenomenon is negatively related to axial length and myopic refraction. It is possible to postulate that increasing of the axial length on this eyes can lead to mechanical stretching of ocular structures, leading to damage to retinal pigmented epithelium (RPE), retinal microvascular network, and endothelial cells. Furthermore, in highly myopic eyes, excessive elongation of the globe and tilting of the optic disc can lead to posterior staphylomas formation and the tilting of the optic disc could lead to alterations in macular and foveal morphology, leading to a change in foveal position that can be found moved mainly in the vertical direction. High axial length is associated with many morphologic changes in the optic nerve and peripapillary region. The axial elongation is associated with the enlargement of the optic nerve head and of the peripapillary scleral tissue. The scleral flange is strongly adherent to the lamina cribrosa and axial-elongation-induced scleral enlargement during eye movements. This condition may lead to thinning of the lamina cribrosa, and it may also be associated with the formation of peripapillary choroidal cavitation. Thinning of lamina cribrosa leads to an alteration between intraocular pressure (optic nerve tissue pressure and cerebrospinal fluid pressure) with a steepening of the translamina cribrosa pressure gradient; this may play a role in the development of the glaucomatous optic neuropathy.

2. Anterior complications in pathologic myopia

2.1 Cataract and pathologic myopia

Three main studies have investigated the connection between cataract formation and high myopia: the Blue Mountains Eye Study and the Beaver Dam study. In the first one, researchers found that there may be a strong connection between the development of posterior polar cataract and myopia that appeared before 20 years. Furthermore, they found a correlation between the level of myopia and posterior subcapsular cataract. High myopia, however, was linked to the formation of all the three types of cataract known [4]. In the Beaver Dam study, researchers confirmed the connection highlighted in other studies between myopia and nuclear cataract [5]. Unlikely, the connection between myopia and age-related cataract is not fully confirmed, while the incidence of PSC and nuclear cataract in myopic eyes appears well established. Also, the distribution of the type of cataract in relation to the axial length of the eye has been investigated; some studies found no connection, while others found a significative direct correlation between AL and the severity of the lens opacity [6]. Eventually, the mechanism that underlies this condition is not fully understood.

2.2 Motility and globe position alterations in high and pathologic myopic patients

High myopia is one of the clinical entities that cause a unilateral proptosis [7], leading to poor cosmesis, motility alterations, and pain. Furthermore, chronic exposition of anterior surface may cause exposition keratopathy. The mechanics of the relationship between axial elongation and myopic proptosis is complex; in its elongation process, the eyeball tends to expand backward and proptosis forward [8].

There is also evidence of a linear correlation between sferic equivalent and proptosis grade. It has been observed that in patients that suffer from strabismus related to high myopia, there is a displacement of the globe from the muscle cone in the space that forms between superior and lateral rectus muscles [9]. Lateral rectus is also inferiorly displaced.

Alterations in motility alterations can also be observed in high myopic eyes; the range of these alterations goes from small angle esotropia with mild reduction of abduction to strabismus fixus. Exotropia and hypotropia can also be seen in these patients. Exodeviations due to a lesser accommodative work are relatively common in myopes.

Strabismus fixus is the latest stage of the abovementioned spectrum; the eye appears fixed in esotropic and hypotropic position; even passive movements in other positions of gaze are impossible. Many theories for that phenomenon have been proposed; one of them is that the displacement of the eyeball already described causes a compression of lateral rectus muscle against the orbital wall. According to other authors, not only lateral rectus muscle can experience this compression, but also superior and medial rectus.

To prove this hypothesis, many MRI studies of the orbit have been performed; some found a displacement of the abovementioned muscles, while others demonstrated a superotemporal prolapse of the elongated posterior portion of the globe, which displaces lateral and superior rectus [10]. High myopic patients with time can also develop diplopia, which is due to esotropia, and hypotropia that is accompanied by limitation of abduction and elevation [11].

Patients that suffer from alterations in motility and position of the globe often have an axial length that is more than 30 mm.

3. Posterior complications in pathologic myopia

3.1 Lacquer cracks

Lacquer cracks are linear breaks of the Bruch's membrane-choriocapillaris complex, which can be found in 4% of subjects with high myopia [12]. The main pathogenetic mechanism is the mechanical stretching of the chorioretinal structures due to scleral elongation [12]. However, according to other studies, their formation could be associated with near vessels perforating the sclera causing the expansion of surrounding scleral tissue [13].

The first clinical presentation usually consists in subretinal hemorrhage, which is a potential sight-threatening condition. Fluoro angiography and indocyanine angiography are important for differential diagnosis with myopic choroidal neovascularization. At the fundus examination, lacquer cracks appear as yellowish-white linear lesions, rarely starry or mixed shapes. Usually, they are located at the posterior pole, and their peripheral formation is unusual [14].

In autofluorescence exam, they appear ipoautofluorescent. Spectral domain optical coherence tomography (SD-OCT) allows studying RPE and Bruch's membrane breaks; "en face" OCT angiography shows avascular bands in choriocapillaris segmentation [12].

Break of Bruch's-choriocapillaris complex leads to near RPE atrophy and fibrotic degeneration. Thus, fluoro angiography shows window-effect hyperfluorescence with no leakage; staining can appear during late phases, especially in fibrotic-evoluted breaks. In those cases, indocyanine angiography shows linear ipocyanescent lesions, which extension results longer than the one appreciable in fluoro angiography exam. Therefore, indocyanine angiography results in a most accurate examination in lacquer crack detection. Breaks on Bruch's-choriocapillaris complex lead to RPE damage and subsequent retina-epithelial "patchy atrophies" and, in 30% of cases, choroidal neovascularization (CNV) [19].

3.2 Chorioretinal atrophy (tessellation, patchy, diffuse)

Choroid thinning and subsequent retinal involvement are typical findings in pathologic myopia. Retinal remodellation seems to be associated with choroidal hypoperfusion due to vascular axial stretching. There are three main atrophy morphologies.

Tessellated fundus is the most common. It consists in multiple linear choroid-RPE thinning, making fundus appear as tiger streaked. Tessellated fundus is a very early manifestation of myopic retinal changes, and it can evolve in other more severe lesions. In fact, it is associated to lacquer crack formation and myopic chorioretinal atrophies.

Patchy atrophy appears as a gray-white lesion with well-defined edges; they can be found on staphyloma edges, near lacquer cracks, or as CNV evolution [15]. Coalescent patchy atrophies can lead to diffuse atrophy; furthermore, they have been described as very important risk factor in CNV formation (20%).

Diffuse atrophy, instead, is a large yellowish-white lesion with no well-defined edges. Usually, it is located in peripapillary zone and its correlation with CNV formation is rare (3.7%). RPE atrophy, patchy ore diffuse, leads to photoreceptor atrophy and their loss of function. Thus, macular or foveal atrophy is responsible of important and irreversible central vision loss. Fluorescein and indocyanine angiographies show hyperfluorescence and hypercyanescence due to window effect. In autofluorescence, atrophy is hypoautofluorescent with mild hyperautofluorescent edges, especially in patchy atrophy.

SD-OCT allows the operator to study the retinal structures involved, measuring progression of lesions over time (**Figure 1**).

The process that can lead to complications due to myopic chorioretinal atrophies is resumed in **Figure 2**.

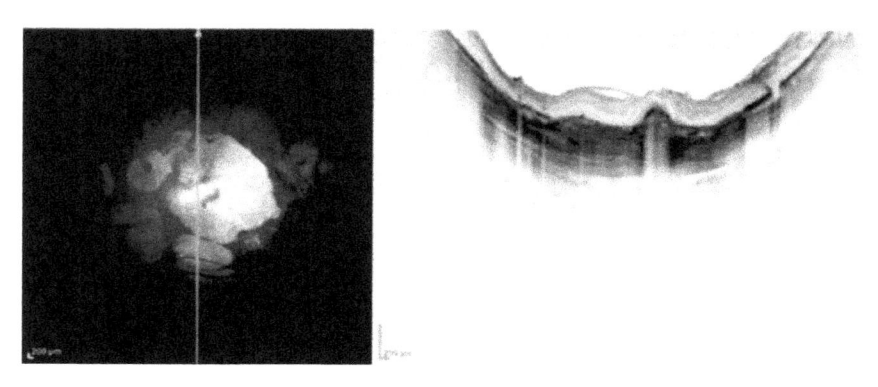

Figure 1.
An OCT scan overlying an area of chorioretinal atrophy: a myopic CNV is also present.

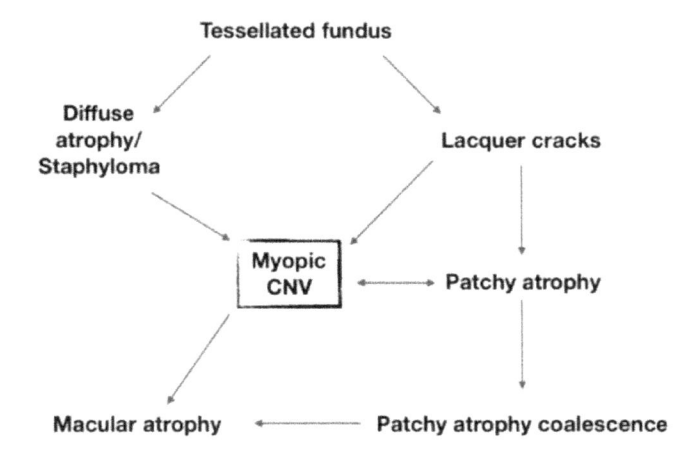

Figure 2.
Myopic chorioretinal atrophies and complications.

3.3 Fuchs' spots

Fuchs' spots are patch-like whitish retinal lesions characterized by a dark pigmented central formation. They are the result of previous myopic CNV and their atrophic evolution with subretinal and intraretinal pigment dispersion. As for patchy atrophies, multiple Fuchs' spots can coalesce forming macular atrophy. Presence of Fuchs' spots in a myopic eye is very important to understand the history of the pathology and its future prognosis [16].

3.4 Myopic CNV

Myopic CNV (mCNV) is found in 5–10% of high myopic eyes. Over time, many environmental and genetic risk factors have been detected. Among the main ones, lacquer cracks (29%), patchy atrophy (20%), female gender, and genetic pro-inflammatory protein expression are important to remember. However, the most important one is history of myopic CNV in the other eye (34%). Very often, mCNVs grow between RPE and neuroepithelium (CNV type 2 or "classic CNV") [17] in the macular region and precisely: 58% foveal and 23% juxtafoveal. Only 19% of mCNVs have extramacular location on the edges of a peripapillary diffuse atrophy (periconus-CNV).

The pathogenesis of mCNVs is still controversial. Their subretinal growth associated to underlying RPE atrophy (75–94% of mCNVs occur on lacquer cracks), together with strong association of choroidal thinning, suggests that an angiogenic stimulus due to choroidal hypoxia could be a plausible pathogenic mechanism, when RPE barrier breaks are present (patchy atrophies and lacquer cracks). Axial length and refractive error, if considered by themselves, do not represent risk factors for mCNVs development [18]. mCNVs growth is asymptomatic until the activation, which leads to rapid reduction of visual acuity with metamorphopsia and scotoma.

On the funduscopic examination, they appear as small grayish spots with pigmented edges; subretinal hemorrhages' and intraretinal exudation are modest.

Fluoro angiography remains the benchmark test for early diagnosis of myopic CNVs, presenting a higher sensitivity than SD-OCT in the detection of early active forms [19].

These lesions appear as hyperfluorescence in the early phases. When active, they show late fluorescein leakage, which is modest when compared to CNV in age-related macular degeneration (AMD). Furthermore, fluoro angiography, when a subretinal hemorrhage occurred, is a fundamental tool in the differential diagnosis between mCNV and Lacquer crack, which typically does not show fluorescein leakage. However, factors such as staining of dye in fibrotic tissue and hemorrhagic blocking defect may reduce the reliability of fluoro angiography exam.

Indocyanine angiography has a better penetration through bleeding, pigment, and exudates; it also allows a more accurate visualization of lacquer cracks. However, sensitivity in identifying CNVs is lower than fluoro angiography. Neovascularizations are shown as inconstant hypercyanescent lesions, sometimes surrounded by a hypocyanescent halo. For these reasons, indocyanine angiography is used only in case of extensive macular hemorrhages and in case of doubtful fluoro angiographic results.

SD-OCT exam is a primary, rapid, and noninvasive test in the diagnosis and follow-up of myopic CNV (**Figure 3**). However, modest exudation and bleeding of active mCNVs can sometimes lead to misdiagnosis on OCT examination. They appear as hyperreflective subretinal formations; signs of exudation (such as intraretinal fluid, retinal thickening, and outer limiting membrane interruption) can be detected only in 48% of cases, while fluorescein leakage is found in 82%. A multimodal approach, combining OCT and fluoro angiography, allows reaching high sensitivity in the diagnosis of myopic CNVs [20].

Overmore, implementation with OCT angiography function allowed us to study the retinal flow in the single tomographic segmentation of the retina, managing to identify 94.1% of mCNVs with a specificity of 93.75%. In "en face" visualization, active CNVs appear as vascular organizations in a typical lacy wheel shape or glomerular pattern, with many anastomoses and thin capillaries, in addition to the typical perilesional dark halo. In the quiescent phase, instead, they assumed the typical aspects of mature neovessels: large caliber and linear course, without anastomosis, with a filiform aspect, or dead tree appearance.

The most effective treatments to date are intravitreal injections of anti-VEGF drugs. While bevacizumab and ranibizumab demonstrated a comparable efficacy, aflibercept allowed the resolution of the CNV with a single administration in 55% of cases, resulting in the best medication for the "result/number of injection" ratio [21].

Photodynamic treatment has been shown to be less effective than ranibizumab; therefore, it is considered as a second choice treatment [22]. Natural evolution of mCNVs consists in a remodellation of the neuroepithelial and pigmented epithelial tissues, leading to the formation of typical Fuchs' spots and patchy atrophies with loss of function of involved retina.

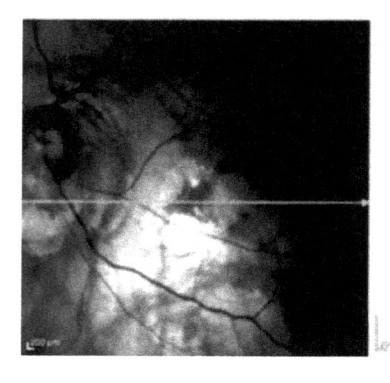

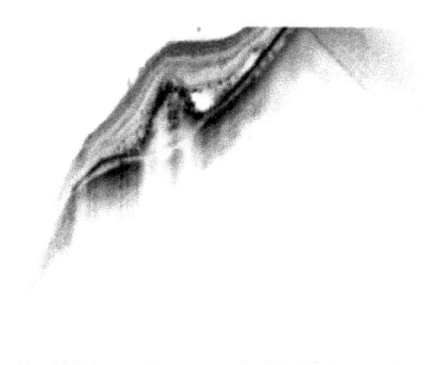

Figure 3.
An OCT scan of a myopic patient showing active myopic CNV.

3.5 Myopic tractional maculopathy (VMT, foveoschisis, macular hole, macular detachment)

The definition of "myopic tractional maculopathy" includes a wide range of pathologies: vitreomacular traction, foveoschisis, and macular hole.

High myopic eyes, with a posterior pole staphyloma, undergo tractional phenomena between stretchable structures and nonelastic structures. To understand the biomechanics underlying these modifications, it is important to consider the physiological adherence of posterior vitreous cortex on the fovea. Furthermore, inner limiting membrane (ILM) and retinal vessels showed a reduced stretching capability compared to choroidal and scleral structures.

The extreme bulbar elongation caused by staphylomas creates axial vitreomacular traction with increased macular thickness; it is usually an asymptomatic condition, or it may lead to metamorphopsia, with preserved or mild altered visual acuity. Axial traction may result in alterations of vitreous body, such as cortical vitreoschisis or posterior vitreous detachment (PVD) (43.2%) with subsequent cellular proliferation and increased risk of epiretinal membrane (ERM) formation.

Progression of staphylomatous bulbar elongation comes up against lower elasticity of retinal internal structures (ILM, retinal vessels, incomplete PVD with vitreoretinal adhesion, ERM), causing an intraretinal cleavage and configuring a foveoschisis (9%) [23]. Cleavage can occur in the inner, outer, or both retinal layers, but more often, it affects the inner limiting membrane. This condition has a variable progression, and some studies demonstrate its stability in 88.4% of cases. However, further progression of axial traction may lead to a detachment of the macular neuroepithelium.

The alteration of posterior pole profile due to the staphyloma, the presence of an ERM, and the incomplete PVD are factors that can lead to the development of tangential traction forces, which, combined with axial traction, can make the foveoschisis evolve into lamellar or full thickness macular holes with important visual acuity impairment. Furthermore, a full-thickness macular hole may cause a rhegmatogenous retinal detachment that can be confined to the macula or also involve the peripheral retina.

Diagnostic strategy of all the clinical presentation analyzed is based on fundus examination and, above all, on the SD-OCT exam. The latter allows a precise characterization of the single vitreoretinal structures involved, through a tomographic study of the bulbar structures. OCT exams also make an accurate, rapid, and noninvasive follow-up possible (**Figure 4**) [24].

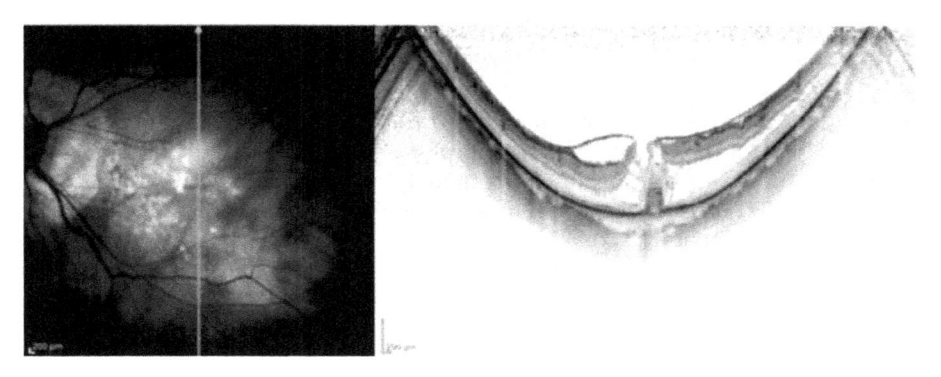

Figure 4.
An OCT of a myopic patient showing a macular pucker and a foveoschisis.

```
        Staphyloma
       (ILM, retinal vessels, VMT)
              │
              ▼
        Foveoschisis
           │      ╲
           │       ╲──▶ Macular Detachment
           ▼       ╱
          FTMH  ◀╱
       (ERM, incomplete DPV)
```

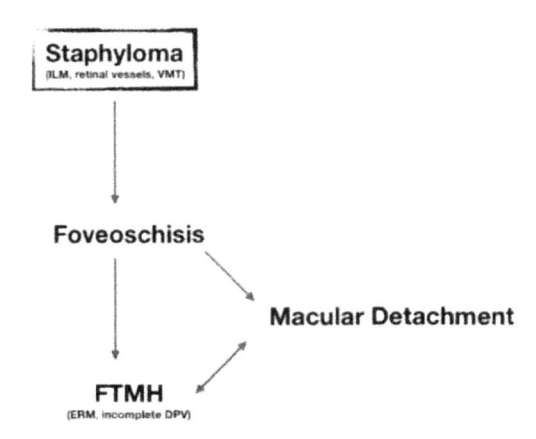

Figure 5.
Myopic tractional maculopathy and complications.

The therapy of myopic tractional maculopathies varies depending on the type of lesion or their combination (foveoschisis, macular hole, macular detachment). Description of surgical procedures is not pertinence of this chapter. In a general way, surgery is the only possible choice and aims at reducing axial and tangential stretching forces. The peeling of ILM and ERM via Pars plana vitrectomy (PPV) is the basis of the resolution of foveoschisis and macular holes [25]. However, sometimes, this approach is not enough, especially if a macular detachment occurred. In these cases, it may be necessary to perform a macular buckle combined or not with PPV.

The pathogenetic process that can lead to the abovementioned complications is resumed in **Figure 5**.

3.6 Retinal detachment

High myopia is the main risk factor for rhegmatogenous retinal detachment; 50% of which, according to some estimates, occurs in myopic patients [26].

Rhegmatogenous retinal detachment is defined as the separation of retinal neuroepithelium from the retinal pigment epithelium following the infiltration of liquefied vitreous material through a full-thickness retinal rupture (tears or holes).

Early vitreal degenerative phenomena leading to syneresis show a peak at young age. Those changes can culminate in a PVD and vitreous liquefaction. This mechanism, typical of myopic eyes, could underlie the higher retinal detachment prevalence. Furthermore, numerous studies have shown a strong association of axial bulbar elongation with various peripheral retinal degenerations, especially with lattice degenerations. These consist in retinal thinning spots with strong vitreous adhesion on the edges, which can exert traction, especially in the presence of PVD. Usually, the vitreous detaches from the retina without causing problems. But, sometimes, the vitreous pulls hard enough to tear the retina in one or more places. Retinal tears can have different shapes and locations. Typically, they are located between equatorial zone and ora-serrata, especially in the upper-temporal quadrant; in over 50% of cases, they appear as circular or oval tears (retinal holes); in the remaining 50%, there are multiple microtears, horseshoe-shaped, and operculated tears [27].

Giant retinal tears are rare and usually associated with bulbar traumas and vitreoretinal proliferation. Overmore, the already mentioned full thickness macular holes can lead to a total retinal detachment in some cases.

Diagnosis of tears and retinal detachment is based on the history and the examination of the fundus oculi. Color peripheral fundus camera and SD-OCT macular scans are often very useful tools. Patients may be asymptomatic or complain of phosphenes and miodesopsias. Standard treatment for retinal tears and lattice degeneration without retinal detachment is argon laser barrage, which has shown to be a very effective prophylactic solution for retinal detachment.

If retinal detachment has already occurred; however, the only therapy is surgery. Ab interno and ab externo approaches are options, but the treatment is delegated to specialistic texts.

3.7 Dome-shaped macula

Features of dome-shaped macula (DMS) are an abnormal profile of the macula that appears convex with an anterior protrusion. Three types of DSM have been described in literature [28]:

- horizontal oval-shaped dome

- vertical oval-shaped dome

- round dome.

DMS can occur in eyes with or without staphyloma and appears related to a localized thinning of the sclera under the dome-shaped macula [29]. This condition can lead to formation of subretinal fluid (SRF) and choroidal neovascularization (CNV). Based on last evidences, the pathologic mechanisms of formation of SRF and CNV could be linked to a similarity of choroid's features between CSCR and only choroid's portion located above the DMS area in high myopic eyes [30]. One of the complications that can occur in eyes with dome-shaped macula is CNV formation, and the types of CNV mostly related to DMS are either typical myopic CNV (i.e., type 2 CNV) or pachychoroid-associated CNV (i.e., type 1 CNV). Another kind of complication related to DMS is the presence of subretinal fluid that causes a chronic serous retinal detachment, which not seems to impair visual function in majority of cases and also shows a certain stability over time. OCT is a crucial technique to observe this condition, because it is almost impossible to detect on standard fundus examination (**Figure 6**). Furthermore, it is crucial to detect the presence of SRF and CNV. Up to date, many treatment approaches such as

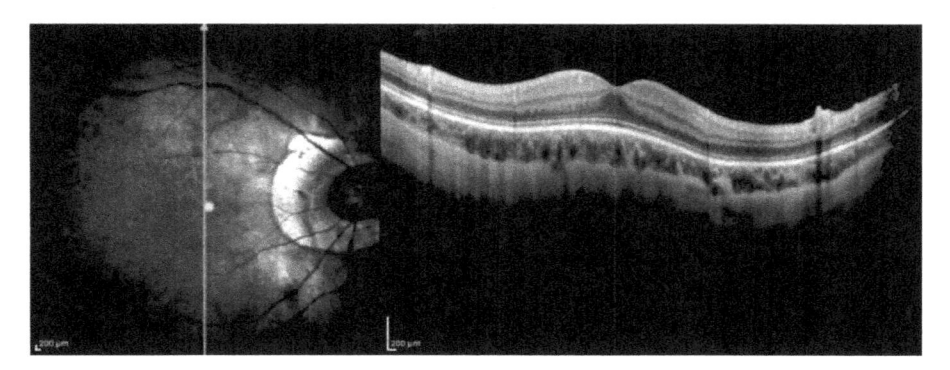

Figure 6.
An OCT of a myopic patient showing a dome-shaped macula.

intravitreal aflibercept, subthreshold laser treatment, PDT, and antimineralocorticoids have been tried to treat SRF associated with DSM, but there is no a definitive one. While representing a potential problem in high myopic eyes, some authors found DMS to be a protective factor for visual function after cataract surgery [31].

3.8 Posterior staphyloma

Posterior staphyloma is defined as "an outpouching of the wall of the eye that has a radius of curvature that is less than the surrounding curvature of the wall of the eye" [32].

Some authors argue that pathologic myopia should not be defined based on axial length but on the presence of staphyloma. An increased presence of staphyloma in eyes exhibits a longer axial length.

According to Curtin, there are many types of staphylomas [33] that can be classified into 10 subcategories. However, also, other classifications have been proposed recently [34]. Methods for detecting staphylomas are OCT, fundus imaging, B mode echography, and 3D magnetic resonance imaging (MRI). Among all, OCT offers the possibility to detect the posterior staphyloma and also to study the morphology of the retinal layers. Interpreting an OCT exam in these cases, it is crucial not to confuse a real staphyloma with a simple scleral backward bowing due to elongation of the eyeball, which is a relatively common finding in high myopic patients. 3D MRI in T2-weighted acquisition perfectly delineates the presence and the type of staphyloma. However, this is not a routine technique and its limits are that it is expensive and that this is not widespread. The presence of a posterior staphyloma can have negative implications on visual outcome, and is also linked to an augmented incidence of other complications such as myopic CNV, myopic macular retinoschisis, and high myopia-associated glaucoma-like defects or glaucomatous optic neuropathy.

4. Low-vision rehabilitation

In many cases, pathologic myopia patients experience an irreversible and deep loss of vision. In such cases, low-vision interventions are useful to allow patients to continue or to improve daily living tasks, independency, and quality of life. Many devices and trainings are available to achieve this goal.

This is an important tool to use in high myopic patients with visual field defects that impair vision, because this is a particularly favorable condition for low-vision correction, mainly because they are used to read at close range of distance.

Low-vision rehabilitation can be approached by many techniques that can be subdivided in two main categories:

a. stimulation techniques (such as visual biofeedback)

b. low-vision aids.

4.1 Stimulation techniques

In general terms, biofeedback is a technique that is used to learn how to control a body function that normally is not under patient's control.

Visual biofeedback can be accomplished by many techniques; in our experience, acoustic biofeedback visual training provides to be the most effective. First of all, it is useful to evaluate patient's retinal sensibility and fixation stability by making a microperimetry (**Figure** 7); this exam allows the examiner to evaluate retinal

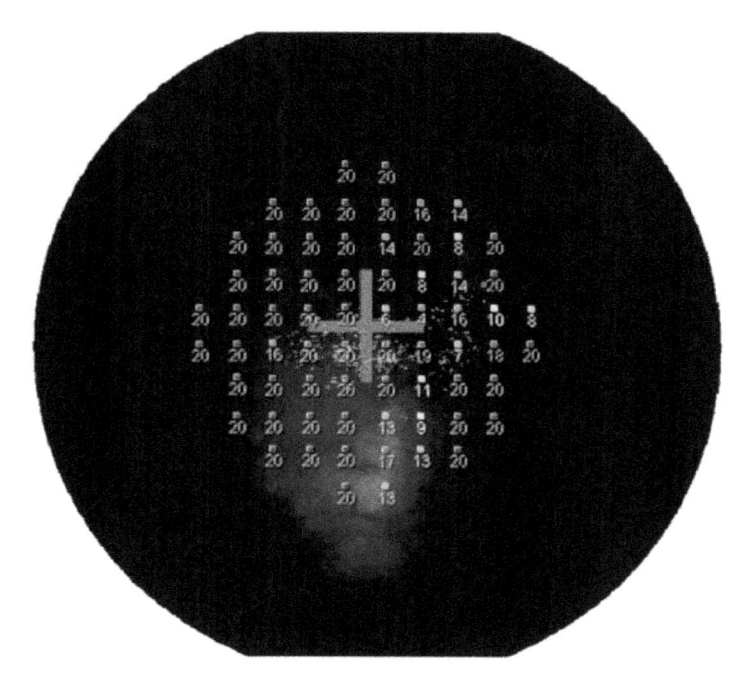

Figure 7.
A microperimetry exam of a high myopic patient who suffered from multiple areas of retinal atrophy and who underwent surgery for retinal detachment, exam prior of acoustic biofeedback training. A threshold of 4-2 strategy with a Goldmann III stimulus was used to perform this exam. An unstable fixation was shown in this patient by means of FUJI classification provided by the machine.

sensitivity in each and every single point of the strategy chosen in a very accurate manner, because the machine presents the light stimulus only when it is perfectly lined with the point to examine by simultaneously analyzing the matching between two or more region of interests (ROIs) chosen by the examiner and the fundus image at that exact moment. This technology, also defined as "fundus-related perimetry," overcomes the main limit of the traditional perimetry: the perfect matching between the stimulus and the point to be stimulated. Then, a fixation stability study using bivariate contour analysis area (BCEA) can be performed. The most important thing in follow-up is to evaluate the fixation stability always in the same manner, since there may be some differences between the one evaluated during microperimetry exam and the one using fixation stability tool, maybe because of the difference in duration between the two exams.

Acoustic visual biofeedback patient is usually done by putting the patient in front of a machine (a microperimeter). The ophthalmologist chooses a point external to the central scotoma to be stimulated and to become a pseudofovea (or stimulates the natural fovea in cases of peripheral visual defects in case of poor fixation stability).

This point is chosen evaluating:

- patient's attitudes and necessities

- retinal sensitivity by means of a microperimetric map

- fixation stability and distribution (bivariate contour ellipse analysis or BCEA)

- distance from the natural fovea.

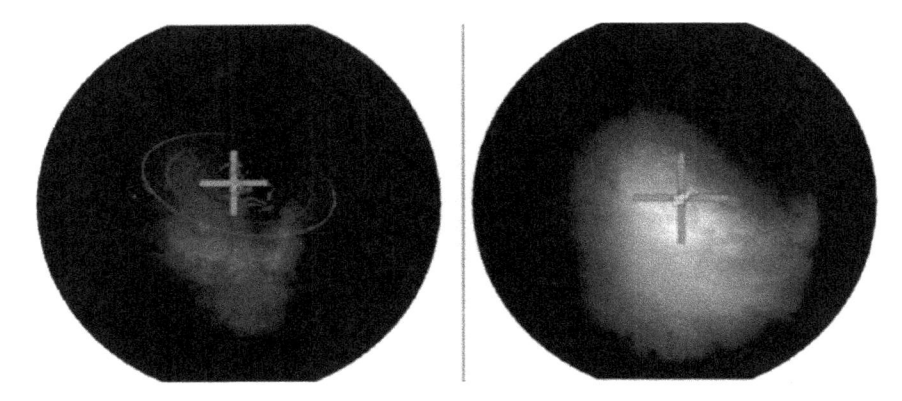

Figure 8.
The fixation stability study (BCEA) of a high myopic patient suffering from a small absolute central scotoma. On the left: before the treatment with acoustic biofeedback; on the right: changes in fixation stability after two treatment of acoustic biofeedback, each of 10 sessions of 10 min. It is possible to appreciate the drastic improvement in fixation stability by means of bivariate contour ellipse analysis.

Regarding last point, it is important to understand that more the distance of the point chosen for stimulation from the natural fovea, the lesser is the outcome to be expected. When the most favorable point to be stimulated is chosen, the patient is asked to firmly look with one eye at a time (in case of rehabilitation of both eyes) to a fixation target inside the microperimeter with the point chosen to be stimulated; during the session, the lesser the distance between the target and the new fixation point chosen, the more continuous the sound emitted by the instrument will be, hence giving the patient a constant control of the retinal point fixing the target. After a training period (usually 10 sessions of 10 min each per eye), the goal is to achieve a constant and stable fixation with the most favorable (in terms of position and residual sensitivity) retinal point other than the fovea previously chosen (**Figure 8**) [35], which is also called pseudofovea, in case of a central scotoma or to achieve a more stable fixation in case of a peripheral defect with a poor fixation stability. All these aspects lead to a better reading performance.

In case of a lesion that leads to a central scotoma, patient's neurovisual system automatically chooses a preferred retinal locus (PRL also known as pseudofovea), which is defined as "one or more circumscribed regions of functioning retina, repeatedly aligned with a visual target for a specified task that may also be used for attention deployment and as the oculomotor reference" [36]. It is also possible to develop two or more PRLs that change accordingly to different tasks. If the ophthalmologist decides to move this PRL using visual biofeedback to a point other than the one automatically set by the patient's brain because he thinks it may be more favorable, it is possible to call it trained retinal locus (TRL). Before starting the treatment, it is absolutely mandatory that the patient has already developed a PRL by itself.

The improvements in fixation stability and PRL relocation observed using acoustic biofeedback technique suggest that a mechanism of cortical reorganization and cortical plasticity may underline those changes [37]. In case of the presence of peripheral visual field defects, a perimetry using 30-2 strategy is useful and can be added to a microperimetry in order to have a more precise evaluation of patient's residual vision.

As already said before, there are two main categories of visual defects that high myopic patients can develop [38]:

- central scotoma (variable in depth, extension, position)

- glaucomatous (if glaucoma develops) or glaucoma-like defects (central and peripheral defects variable in depth, extension, position).

It is well known that patients affected by absolute central scotoma from other kinds of maculopathies may benefit from visual biofeedback training. Highly myopic patients develop macular complications that can lead to this kind of defect, hence making this kind of therapy beneficial also to those patients. Due to the risk of developing glaucoma and/or glaucoma-like defects as mentioned above, acoustic biofeedback can be a useful technique in the visual rehabilitation of those patients. Many studies proved the efficacy of this technique in advanced glaucomatous damage in improving fixation stability and visual performances in patients with glaucoma.

4.2 Visual aids

Visual aids are tools (optical or technological) that may improve visual performances in low-vision patients such as high myopic patient in which visual defects have already developed.

For didactic purposes, we will divide them into three main categories:

a. for distance and intermediate vision

b. for near vision and reading

c. field enhancement.

4.2.1 For distance and intermediate vision

Telescopic systems are the hallmark of this category, and they work by producing magnification. There are two main kinds of telescopes: the Galilean and the Keplerian ones. A Galilean telescope works by coupling a convex lens (object) and a concave lens (ocular) [39]; the image produced is real and erect. A Keplerian telescope is made by the combination of two lenses: a convex lens, which is closest to the object (the ocular lens) and a convex lens (the objective lens), which is closest to the eye and has less dioptric power than the first one. The distance between the two lenses is the result of the sum of their focal length. Since the image produced is inverted, a prism is required in order to reverse it. This kind of telescope has more wide field of view, less aberrations, and a better image quality than Galilean ones, but they are a little bit less comfortable since they are heavier and often more expensive. In contrast, Galilean telescope is lighter, cheaper, and shorter, making them handier for the patient. Telescopes are very effective for distance tasks, but they present some problems. They have a steep learning curve because of the restricted field of view, and the learning process is a struggle because of the distortion provided on space and objects. Telescopes are available in many forms such as hand held, spectacle mounted (**Figure 9**), and clip-on. They may also have fixed or variable focus. Spectacle mounted is obtained by cutting an hole in the spectacle lenses and inserting the telescope; this one can be placed at the center of the lens or higher than the center; this position is particularly useful since the patient uses the center of his lens for most of the time and can look through the telescope placed in the upper part of his spectacles only when he needs to magnify some distant object (such as, for example, traffic signs) [40].

4.2.2 For near vision and reading

Microscopic systems are high dioptric positive power lens that work by reducing focal length. There are many solutions that use this technology. Handheld magnifiers are variable positive power lens with handle, aspheric or biconvex, in various dioptric power and magnification, whether illuminated or not. High positive power lens are

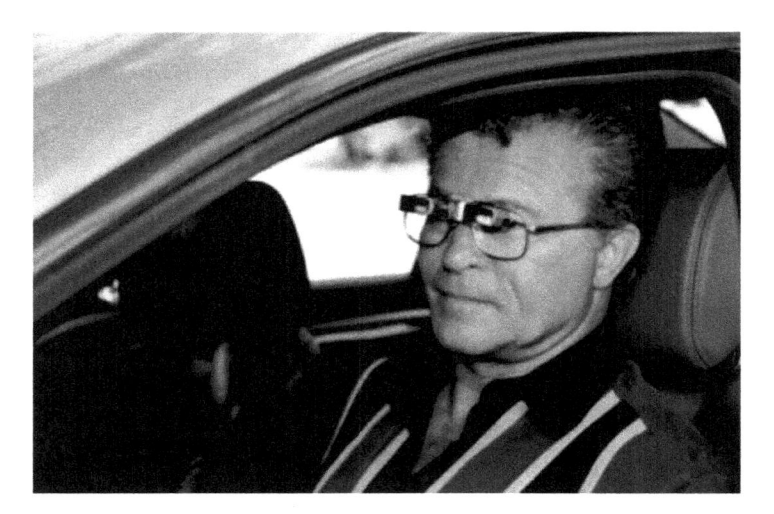

Figure 9.
A patient driving using binocular telescopes mounted on top of the spectacle lenses.

available also as pocket magnifiers. Bar magnifiers are variable length bars able to magnify a text by sliding upon it. They are available in different dioptric powers (hence different magnification) and can be illuminated or not. Another option is high positive dioptric power lens spectacle mounted. However, they pose some struggling: the higher the power, the lesser the distance between the text/object and lens; the higher the power the, higher the convergence required to the patient. Binocular microscopic systems (also known as prismatic hypercorrective) are spectacle-mounted hypercorrective lens, which consist in two positive lenses and two prisms that are calculated based on the power of the positive lens; this kind of glass is found in various amount of magnification and dioptric power (usually from +3.00 to 16.00 dpt). The higher the magnification, the higher the difficulty of the patient to adapt to this kind of lowvision aid. The aim of the use of the prisms is to reduce the amount of the convergence required to the patient due to the use of the reduced working distance, hence reducing discomfort from prolonged tasks as for example reading a book. As we said before, one of the key mechanisms to improve reading performance in low vision is magnification [41]. Many electronic devices exist to accomplish this job; one of them is closed circuit television (CCTV). These systems are often reserved to visually impaired people with severe low vision in which the magnification needed to be able to read or to do it more fluently should be as high that optic systems would not be comfortable and usable [42] to. These are called CCTV to differentiate them from broadcast television. This system can also be useful for writing. Behind the lens of the CCTV camera, there is an image sensor, which is equivalent to a retina. This lens system refracts light beams reflected from an object and focuses them on the plate to become an image.

Based on information sheets of American Foundation for the Blind (AFB), a CCTV (**Figure 10**) must have these characteristics:

- video camera mounted on a fixed stand (some models have optics able to provide zoom while others not; some have autofocus while others not)

- TV or monitor from 5″ to 20″

- positive magnification from 2× to 60× (but also even more)

- polarity inversion (from black-white to white-black)

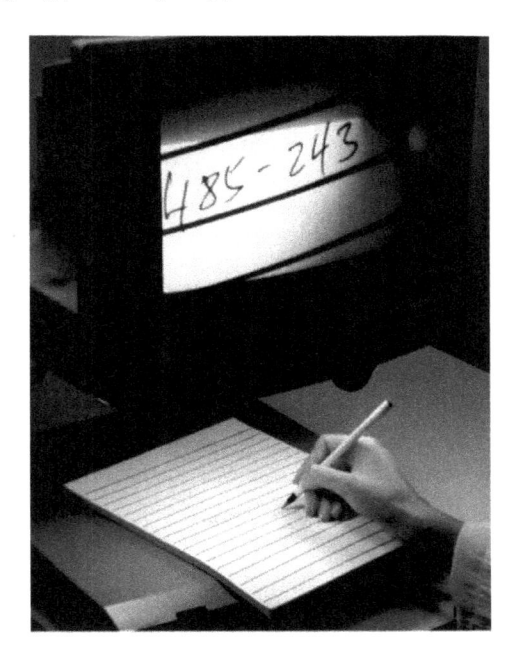

Figure 10.
A CCTV used for writing.

- focus, contrast, and brightness controls

- table that moves on an X-Y direction.

Many kinds of CCTV systems are available in the market; the main difference is between portable CCTV and table-mounted systems. The first one is extremely useful for children with low vision, because they can be used at home and at school, for leisure and for studying. Recently, there has been some evidence that these kinds of devices may be more effective than optical devices in improving reading speed [43].

Portable systems are usually composed by a camera with optics able to provide a variable amount of zoom and hence magnification, an LCD screen (usually small and in most cases within 10″), and an handle to be held by the patient. They are designed to be portable: in most cases, they can be placed in the pocket, or in the case of largest ones in a bag. They are useful in daily activities such as drugs assumption, reading letters, buying products in drugstore, etc. In our experience, however, they are most useful in case of low-vision patients with a nonsevere low vision that allows the patients a certain level of self-sufficiency. Also, portable video magnifiers without screen included exist.

An example of this technology is the mouse video magnifier. It consists in a camera mounted on a mouse that slides above the text, which is projected on a screen. The screen is not included; this device must be connected to a monitor, a PC, or a TV to be used. In some cases, these products are provided with computer software that allows capture of images on the patient's PC.

4.2.3 Other kinds of devices

Many braille systems exist on the market. One of them is the braille printer, which works like a normal printer with the difference that it prints braille text onto a thick paper. Those devices are usually linked to a computer equipped with braille

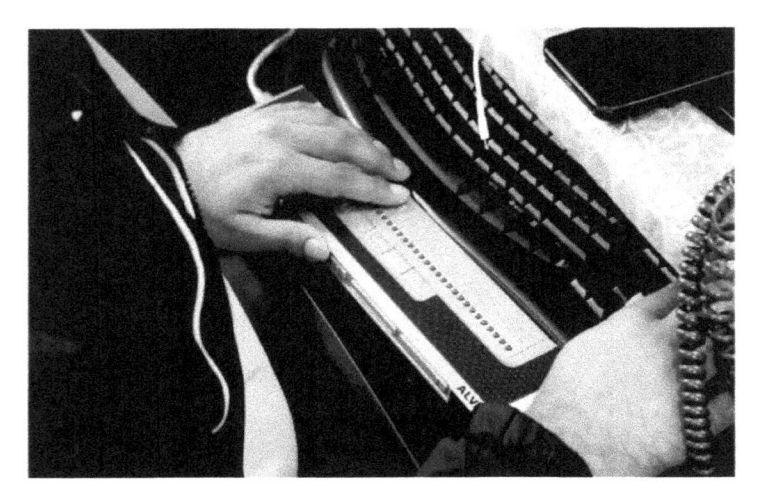

Figure 11.
A braille display.

translator software that converts a text from a language into a braille text. This text is then embossed into a thick paper with a braille printer [44].

Braille displays (**Figure 11**) are special displays made of special materials (metals or plastics). They instantly translate the text into braille that is appearing on the computer, and they change with the scrolling of the text on the PC screen. They are usually placed under the PC keyboard. Also portable note takers exit, making patients able to take notes via a keyboard in braille; the system is then able to recall and read them via voice activation. A braille writer is very similar to a standard typewriter, with the difference that its keyboard is made in braille. It instantly embosses letters on a thick paper. System based on optical character recognition (OCR) is made of a camera, which scans the text; this is then read by the system itself via a synthetized voice. Many OCR systems offer special features such as storage of the texts acquired, research of words, and chapters of the text. The advantage of these systems is that they are not dependent on a PC for working. Many OCR apps are now available, hence making this technology more widespread [45].

Audiobooks are another useful option in low-vision patients of pathologic myopia. Almost any of the best-known novels can be found in audiobook format, in which a voice reads the texts for the listeners. Many low-vision societies make audiobooks available and also apps for new devices such as that found in tablets.

4.2.4 Household, personal, and other independent living products

In this category, all the devices that improve patient's self-sufficiency, safety, and quality of life are included. As many of them exist, we will cite only the best known: vibrating-, braille and talking watches, talking blood pressure- and glucose meters, talking thermometers, weighted eating utensil fork, talking kitchen scale, cut-resistant gloves, talking microwave, labeling systems, object locators, etc.

4.2.5 Field enhancement

As we already said, pathologic myopic patients are at risk to develop glaucoma and optic neuropathies. Patients can also develop ring-shaped scotomas even if the patient is not affected by glaucoma. However, when this pathology is present, one of the visual field alterations that a patient suffering from glaucoma can experience is the restriction of the peripheral visual field up to the development of a tubular field of view. In the abovementioned cases, field enhancers are useful. There are many tools that can act as field expanders such as reverse telescopes, minifiers, and prisms. Minifiers act by "miniaturizing the space" in order to maximize the portion of this one that can be seen into a tubular visual field. There are many powers of miniaturization on the market; best known are 0.25× and 0.5×. They can be found as handheld, clip-on, or spectacle mounted. Reverse telescopes are Galilean or Keplerian telescopes used by the object lens and not by the ocular lens; in this way, a minification of the space is obtained in order to fit a restricted visual field and the power of minification is equal to the power of the telescope [46].

Minification devices are a useful help only in static situation, because patient is not able to use them while walking since he perceives many aberrations and a very restricted visual field. Prisms combined in a field expanding channel lens are also an option in such cases [47]. This spectacle lens is made of two lateral prisms of 12 pd and an inferior one of 8 pd; a central nonprismatic lens, which has the dioptric power of the distance vision prescription, is also present. Prisms work only in position of gaze different than the primary. This lens can be built and used for peripheral defects even more than 20°.

5. Conclusions

High myopia, defined as refractive error of at least −6.00D and/or an axial length of 26.5 mm or more, can lead to many morphological changes in the eyeball that can cause development of complications. World is facing a rapid rise in high myopia and pathologic myopia incidence, and some areas of the globe show a more rapid increase in this trend than other ones, such as Asian regions. In such areas, the incidence rate can also reach 80–90% of children and young adults in school age. Major risk factors in myopia progression are intensive education and limited time outdoors. It is estimated that this percentage and the magnitude of myopic shift will rise in the future because of the rising educational pressure and needs especially in developing countries. The constant rising in the amount of time spent using high-tech devices worldwide such as tablets and smartphone and its use by children represents an adjunctive risk factor. These evidences produce a worrying outline for the future, because early onset of myopia in childhood is associated with high myopia in adult life. Prevention in such cases can count on interventions on school system, favoring open air activities if possible, and children's lifestyle modifications [48], spending more time outside and reducing the time spent with electronic devices. Recently, many clinical trials investigated the role of pharmacologic therapy with atropine 0.01% eye drops and orthokeratology [49] in slowing the progression of myopia in children and young individuals with good results.

Studies estimated that by 2050, half of the global population (5 billion people) would be myopic and 25% of those (1 billion) would be considered highly myopic (>−5D), making it a serious problem for healthcare systems and governments facing the rise in healthcare expenditure, because such patients have a greater need of care and assistive devices, low-vision interventions, and a greater impact of the disease on their work productivity, eventually quitting work and hence increasing the costs of this pathology. In our opinion, prevention of high myopia by reducing near work when possible and stimulating open-air activities for children is essential; we also think that atropine drops will be an useful tool for reducing the rising in incidence of myopia in children. For senior individuals affected by high myopia, a comprehensive ophthalmologic assessment with OCT exam, each 6–12 months, depending on the degree of myopia, is in our opinion crucial to be able to act promptly in case of onset of complications related to high myopia.

As above mentioned, when complications due to high myopia occur, we talk about pathologic myopia. Many complications can develop, and their treatment can count mainly on surgery and anti-VEGF therapy. When treatment is not possible or after this in order to boost and maximize the visual recovery, ophthalmologist can recur to visual rehabilitation strategies. These can count into two main categories of tools: visual stimulation and visual aids. Acoustic biofeedback is one of the most effective techniques in order to stimulate visual system. First of all, it is mandatory to analyze the characteristics of the visual field defects that are affecting the patient. Two types of defects can occur in such patients: central scotomas (of various shape, size, and depth) and peripheral defects. The two can also occur simultaneously in various combinations. Then, in case of a central defect, after analyzing patient's retinal sensitivity and fixation stability with a microperimetry, if the patient has already developed a preferred retinal locus (PRL or pseudofovea) by itself, it is possible to stimulate this one if it is in a favorable position in order to boost fixation stability or to choose a new point to relocate the PRL in a position that the physician considers more favorable for the patient because of a better residual retinal sensitivity. A PRL is a point that the patient with a central scotoma uses to fixate object, as a "substitute" of the natural impaired fovea. This point is chosen considering patient's expectations, attitudes, activities and the residual sensitivity microperimetric map of the patient and the distance that the point candidate to be stimulated from the natural fovea. It means that for a better outcome it would be better to choose a point with the best residual retinal sensitivity not too far from the natural fovea if possible. Acoustic biofeedback is a technique that trains the patient relocating the PRL to a more useful position; when a point to become the new PRL is chosen by the examiner, during the acoustic biofeedback session, a beep is produced by the machine (microperimeter), and it becomes more continuous as the point to be stimulated gets closer to the center of the fixation target on the machine, hence training the patient to use the point set by the ophthalmologist. This one guides the patient during the whole session, giving him instructions where to move his gaze to match the trained PRL and the center of the fixation point of the machine. A typical acoustic biofeedback rehabilitation protocol is composed of 10 sessions of 10 min each, typically one session per week. However, it can be repeated if necessary. In case of a peripheral defect alone, acoustic biofeedback can be useful if an unstable fixation is present in order to stimulate the fixation point and make it more stable. Visual aid use can also benefit of a more stable fixation; they are available for distance and intermediate-near vision. For distance vision, the most popular devices are telescopes, Galilean, and Keplerian ones. They ideally "approach" far items to the observer by magnifying them. They can be monocular or binocular, clip-on, spectacle mounted, and handheld. For near vision, microscopic systems are available; they are high dioptric positive power lens that work by reducing focal length. There are many solutions that use this technology: handheld magnifiers, bar magnifiers, positive overcorrection of near prescription, visolettes, and prismatic hypercorrective are available in various spherical powers and so in various magnification power. Electronic aids for near vision are available, with portable and fixed CCTV being the mainstay of the category. Other solutions are also available such as braille systems (displays, printers, note takers), household, personal and other independent living products (for example, braille and talking watches, talking blood pressure and glucose meters, etc.), OCR systems, and audiobooks. Many recent apps for aided mobility, OCR, etc., have been placed on the market. In patients with peripheral visual field defects, field enhancement systems are very useful. Reversed telescopes and field expanding channel lens represent the mainstay of this category.

Conflict of interest

Enzo Maria Vingolo, Giuseppe Napolitano, and Lorenzo Casillo declare that they have no conflict of interest.

Notes/thanks/other declarations

Authors would like to thank and dedicate this chapter to all the staffs of ophthalmology department in our hospital. You all are great!

Author details

Enzo Maria Vingolo*, Giuseppe Napolitano and Lorenzo Casillo
Department of Medical-Surgical Sciences and Biotechnologies,
U.O.C. Ophthalmology, Sapienza University of Rome, Terracina, Italy

*Address all correspondence to: enzomaria.vingolo@uniroma1.it

IntechOpen

© 2019 The Author(s). Licensee IntechOpen. This chapter is distributed under the terms of the Creative Commons Attribution License (http://creativecommons.org/licenses/by/3.0), which permits unrestricted use, distribution, and reproduction in any medium, provided the original work is properly cited. (cc) BY

References

[1] Chang SW, Tsai IL, Hu FR, et al. The cornea in young myopic adults. The British Journal of Ophthalmology. 2001;**85**:916-920

[2] Ortiz S et al. Relationships between central and peripheral corneal thickness in different degrees of myopia. Journal of Optometry. 2014;**7**(1):44-50

[3] Ikuno Y, Tano Y. Retinal and choroidal biometry in highly myopic eyes with spectral-domain optical coherence tomography. Investigative Ophthalmology & Visual Science. 2009;**50**:3876-3880

[4] Lim R, Mitchell P, Cumming RG. Refractive associations with cataract: The Blue Mountains Eye Study. Investigative Ophthalmology & Visual Science. 1999;**40**(12):3021-3026

[5] Lee KE, Klein BE, Klein R, et al. Changes in refraction over 10 years in an adult population: The Beaver Dam Eye study. Investigative Ophthalmology & Visual Science. 2002;**43**:2566-2571

[6] Pan C-W, Boey PY, Cheng C-Y, et al. Myopia, axial length, and age-related cataract: The Singapore Malay Eye Study. Investigative Ophthalmology & Visual Science. 2013;**54**(7):4498-4502. DOI: 10.1167/iovs.13-12271

[7] Satchi K, McNab AA. Orbital decompression in the treatment of proptosis due to high axial myopia. Ophthalmic Plastic & Reconstructive Surgery. 2010;**26**(6):420-425

[8] Chen M, Zhou XT, Xue AQ, Wang QM, et al. Myopic proptosis and the associated changes in axial components of the eye. Zhonghua Yan Ke Za Zhi. 2007;**43**(6):525-529

[9] Yamaguchi M, Yokoyama T, Shiraki K. Surgical procedure for correcting globe dislocation in higly myopic strabismus. American Journal of Ophthalmology. 2010;**149**:341-346

[10] Yokoyama T. Ocular motility abnormalities. In: Spaide R, Ohno-Matsui K, Yannuzzi L, editors. Pathologic Myopia. New York, NY: Springer; 2014

[11] Taylor R, Whale K, Raines M. The Heavy Eye Phenomenon: Orthoptic and ophthalmic characteristics. German Journal of Ophthalmology. 1995;**4**:252-255

[12] Liu C-F, Liu L, Lai C-C, et al. Multimodal imaging including spectral-domain optical coherence tomography and confocal near-infrared reflectance for characterization of lacquer cracks in highly myopic eyes. Eye (London, England). 2014;**28**(12):1437-1445. DOI: 10.1038/eye.2014.221. Epub 2014 Sep 19

[13] Querques G, Corvi F, Balaratnasingam C, et al. Lacquer cracks and perforating scleral vessels in pathologic myopia: A possible causal relationship. American Journal of Ophthalmology. 2015;**160**(4):759-766

[14] Suga M, Shinohara K, Ohno-Matsui K. Lacquer cracks observed in peripheral fundus of eyes with high myopia. International Medical Case Reports Journal. 2017;**10**:127-130. DOI: 10.2147/IMCRJ.S131545

[15] Ohno-Matsui K, Jonas JB, Spaide RF. Macular Bruch membrane holes in highly myopic patchy chorioretinal atrophy. American Journal of Ophthalmology. 2016;**166**:22-28. DOI: 10.1016/j.ajo.2016.03.019. Epub 2016 Mar 24

[16] Soubrane G. Choroidal neovascularization in pathologic myopia: recent developments in diagnosis and treatment. Survey of Ophthalmology. 2008;**53**(2):121-138

[17] Miyata M et al. Detection of myopic choroidal neovascularization using optical coherence tomography angiography. American Journal of Ophthalmology. 2016;**165**:108-114

[18] Wong TY, Ohno-Matsui K, Leveziel N, et al. Myopic choroidal neovascularisation: Current concepts and update on clinical management. British Journal of Ophthalmology. 2015;**99**:289-296

[19] Leveziel N, Caillaux V, Bastuji-Garin S, et al. Angiographic and optical coherence tomography characteristics of recent myopic choroidal neovascularization. American Journal of Ophthalmology. 2013;**155**(5):913-919. DOI: 10.1016/j.ajo.2012.11.021. Epub 2013 Jan 23

[20] Milani P, Massacesi A, Moschini S, et al. Multimodal imaging and diagnosis of myopic choroidal neovascularization in Caucasians. Clinical Ophthalmology. 2016;**10**:1749-1757. DOI: 10.2147/OPTH.S108509

[21] Ikuno Y, Ohno-Matsui K, Wong TY, et al. Intravitreal aflibercept injection in patients with myopic choroidal neovascularization: The MYRROR study. Ophthalmology. Jun 2015;**122**(6):1220-1227. DOI: 10.1016/j.ophtha.2015.01.025. Epub 2015 Mar 4

[22] Wolf S, Balciuniene VJ, Laganovska G, et al. RADIANCE: A randomized controlled study of ranibizumab in patients with choroidal neovascularization secondary to pathologic myopia. Ophthalmology. 2014;**121**(3):682-92.e2. DOI: 10.1016/j.ophtha.2013.10.023. Epub 2013 Dec 8

[23] Baba T, Ohno-Matsui K, Futagami S. Prevalence and characteristics of foveal retinal detachment without macular hole in high myopia. American Journal of Ophthalmology. 2003;**135**(3):338-342

[24] Gómez-Resa M, Burés-Jelstrup A, Mateo C. Myopic traction maculopathy. In: Microincision Vitrectomy Surgery. Vol. 54. Karger Publishers; 2014. pp. 204-212

[25] Mii M, Matsuoka M, Matsuyama K, et al. Favorable anatomic and visual outcomes with 25-gauge vitrectomy for myopic foveoschisis. Clinical Ophthalmology. 2014;**8**:1837-1844. DOI: 10.2147/OPTH.S67619

[26] Steel D. Retinal detachment. BMJ Clinical Evidence. 2014;**2014**:0710

[27] Alimanović-Halilović E. Correlation between refraction level and retinal breaks in myopic eye. Bosnian Journal of Basic Medical Sciences. 2008;**8**(4):346-349. DOI: 10.17305/bjbms.2008.2895. ISSN 1840-4812

[28] Caillaux V, Gaucher D, Gualino V, et al. Morphologic characterization of dome-shaped macula in myopic eyes with serous macular detachment. American Journal of Ophthalmology. 2013;**156**(5):958-967.e1. DOI: 10.1016/j.ajo.2013.06.032. Epub 2013 Aug 20

[29] Ng DS, Cheung CY, Luk FO, et al. Advances of optical coherence tomography in myopia and pathologic myopia. Eye (London, England). 2016;**30**(7):901-916. DOI: 10.1038/eye.2016.47. Epub 2016 Apr 8

[30] Viola F, Dell'Arti L, Benatti E, et al. Choroidal findings in dome-shaped macula in highly myopic eyes: A longitudinal study. American Journal of Ophthalmology. 2015;**159**(1):44-52. DOI: 10.1016/j.ajo.2014.09.026. Epub 2014 Sep 22

[31] Zhu X, He W, Zhang S, et al. Dome-shaped macula: A potential protective factor for visual acuity after cataract surgery in patients with high myopia. The British Journal of Ophthalmology. 2019. pii: bjophthalmol-2018-313279. DOI: 10.1136/bjophthalmol-2018-313279. [Epub ahead of print]

[32] Spaide RF. Staphyloma: Part 1. In: Spaide RF, Ohno-Matsui K, Yannuzzi LA, editors. Pathologic Myopia. New York, NY: Springer; 2014. pp. 167-176

[33] Curtin BJ. The posterior staphyloma of pathologic myopia. Transactions of the American Ophthalmological Society. 1977;**75**:67-86

[34] Ohno-Matsui K. Proposed classification of posterior staphylomas based on analyses of eye shape by three-dimensional magnetic resonance imaging and wide-field fundus imaging. Ophthalmology. 2014;**121**:1798-1809

[35] Vingolo EM, Napolitano G, Fragiotta S. Microperimetric biofeedback training: Fundamentals, strategies and perspectives. Frontiers in Bioscience (Scholar Edition). 2018;**10**(1):48-64

[36] Crossland MD, Engel SA, Legge GE. The preferred retinal locus in macular disease: Toward a consensus definition. Retina. 2011;**31**:2109-2114. DOI: 10.1097/IAE.0b013e31820d3fba

[37] Dilks DD, Julian JB, Peli E, et al. Reorganization of visual processing in age-related macular degeneration depends on foveal loss. Optometry and Vision Science. 2014;**91**(8):e199-e206

[38] Ohno-Matsui K, Shimada N, Yasuzumi K, et al. Long-term development of significant visual field defects in highly myopic eyes. American Journal of Ophthalmology 2011;**152**(2):256-265.e1. DOI: 10.1016/j.ajo.2011.01.052. Epub 2011 Jun 12

[39] Vasconcelos G, Fernandes LC. Low-Vision Aids. 2015. Retrieved from: https://www.aao.org/disease-review/low-vision-aids

[40] Chun R, Cucuras M, Jay WM. Current perspectives of bioptic driving in low vision. Neuroophthalmology. 2016;**40**(2):53-58. DOI: 10.3109/01658107.2015.1134585

[41] Legge GE. Reading digital with low vision. Visible Language. 2016;**50**(2):102-125

[42] Burggraaff MC, van Nispen RMA, Knol DL, Ringens PJ, van Rens GHMB. Randomized controlled trial on the effects of CCTV training on quality of life, depression, and adaptation to vision loss. Investigative Ophthalmology & Visual Science. 2012;**53**(7):3645-3652. DOI: 10.1167/iovs.11-9226

[43] Virgili G, Acosta R, Bentley SA, et al. Reading aids for adults with low vision. Cochrane Database of Systematic Reviews. 2018;**4**:CD003303. DOI: 10.1002/14651858.CD003303.pub4

[44] Kalia A, Hopkins R, Jin D, et al. Perception of tactile graphics: Embossings versus cutouts. Multisensory Research. 2014;**27**(2):111-125

[45] Cutter M, Manduchi R. Improving the accessibility of mobile OCR apps via interactive modalities. ACM Transactions on Accessible Computing. 2017;**10**(4):11

[46] Krefman RA. Reversed telescopes on visual efficiency scores in field-restricted patients. American Journal of Optometry and Physiological Optics. 1981;**58**:159-162

[47] Apfelbaum H, Peli E. Tunnel vision prismatic field expansion: Challenges and requirements. Translational Vision Science & Technology. 2015;**4**(6):8. DOI: 10.1167/tvst.4.6.8

[48] Morgan IG, French AN, Ashby RS, et al. The epidemics of myopia: Aetiology and prevention. Progress in Retinal and Eye Research. 2018;**62**:134-149

[49] Leo SW. Current approaches to myopia control. Current Opinion in Ophthalmology. 2017;**28**(3):267-275

Chapter 7

Reduction of Myopia Burden and Progression

Sangeethabalasri Pugazhendhi, Balamurali Ambati and Allan A. Hunter

Abstract

Myopia is a significant worldwide public health concern, and its prevalence is drastically increasing in recent years. It was once viewed as a benign refractive error, but is now one of the leading causes of blindness and is associated with numerous ocular diseases, which makes it crucial to develop viable treatment options to adequately correct the refractive error and to halt the disease progression. The treatment of myopia can be classified into three groups: optical, pharmacological, and surgical management, which are aimed at adjusting to the refractive error and reducing the axial elongation. The conventional treatment modalities for myopia, such as single vision glasses, correct the refractive error and improve visual quality of life, but do not affect myopia progression or axial elongation. The newer and various myopic interventions including spectacle corrections, contact lens corrections, pharmacological treatments and surgical corrections, hold great potential for adequate disease control to improve the quality of life, reduce myopia burden, and preserve the ocular health.

Keywords: myopia, refractive error, axial elongation, single vision lenses, multifocal lenses, rigid gas permeable contact lenses, soft bifocal contact lens, orthokeratology, atropine, pirenzepine, anti-hypoxic drugs

1. Introduction

Myopia is a refractive condition of the eye that has globally affected 1.89 billion people worldwide, and projected to affect 2.56 billion people by the year 2020 [1]. Over the past few decades, the prevalence of myopia in Asia has increased dramatically affecting as much as 80–90% of the pediatric Asian population, and 25–50% of the American and European population [2].

Refractive development in early ocular growth is an intricate and continuous process. At birth, there is a high prevalence of large refractive errors in newborn infants due to mismatch between the axial length and the focal length of its optics [3–5]. As the newborn matures, the eye develops in size and refracting power in a rapid fashion to attain an ideal refractive state in early childhood. This physiological process is known as emmetropization [5–7]. Coordination between axial length and optical components will allow for the images of distal objects to focus on the retina, rather than in front or behind it [5]. Interruption of this homeostatic process of ocular growth results in the development of refractive error. The disorder manifests in early childhood and progresses at an average of 0.5D every year until stabilizing during adolescence [8–10].

It was once considered a mere refractive error, but myopia is now often associated with a multitude of ocular diseases such as retinal detachment, glaucoma, cataract and chorioretinal abnormalities [11]. Therefore, in recent years, the focus of myopia research has been on halting the progression to decrease the risk of associated future ocular diseases.

This chapter focuses on the mechanics of the various treatment methods including optical, pharmacological and surgical strategies, for precise control of myopia. The goal of such treatment methods is to reduce both personal and societal burden, as well as prevent disease progression such as worsening refractions, axial length and overall ocular health.

2. Treatment of myopia

2.1 Optical management

2.1.1 Spectacle correction

While potential optical strategies are investigated for adequate myopia control, the visual outcomes of Single Vision Lenses (SVLs) are used as control for efficacy comparison. Single vision lenses (SVLs) have universally been utilized by ophthalmologists and optometrists for correction of refractive error. With periodic monitoring, the spectacle prescription is often adjusted to correct the increasing refractive error. The growth of the eye is regulated by visual signals, which are manipulated and controlled by the power of the spectacle lens [5]. By regulating the refractive error of the cornea and the axial length of the eye, SVLs emulate the eye's innate process of emmetropization by allowing the eye to focus the rays on the retina [5, 12].

While visual outcomes are improved, SVLs do not interrupt the myopia progression or axial length elongation. Though clinically insignificant, evidence from animal studies suggest compensatory eye growth in spectacle induced emmetropization [13, 14]. Since SVLs alter the refractive error but does not reduce progression or axial elongation, studies have investigated on alternate optical correction methods, such as under-correction of refractive error.

Animal studies have postulated that under-correction of the refractive error reduces the mean change in refractive error, in comparison to fully-corrected SVLs. Hence, some clinicians advocate for under-corrected SVLs in an attempt to reduce the axial growth and prevent further myopia progression. It is theorized that modest under-correction of SVLs by 0.5–0.75D reduces the accommodative stimulus and consequently the blur drive for near work accommodation [15, 16]. However, studies have demonstrated contradicting results.

The pilot randomized study performed by Chung et al. compared the effects of under correction versus full correction on Hong Kong Chinese children. The study demonstrated that myopia progression was slightly greater in patients with under-correction in comparison to full correction, with 0.5 and 0.35D, respectively [17]. Similar results were obtained by study conducted by Adler et al., which showed 0.66 versus 0.55D for patients with under-correction and full correction, respectively [18]. Both studies concluded that myopic defocus through under-correction slightly increased the rate of myopia progression. While SVLs attend to the refractive error and vision complaints of the child, it does not have a protective role on the health and growth of the eye.

As an alternative to SVLs, multifocal lenses have gained popularity for use in slowing or halting the progression of myopia and axial elongation of the eye. It is believed that these lenses decrease the rate of myopia progression by reducing accommodation effort and hyperopic defocus. A relatively newer version of the multifocal lenses is Progressive Addition Lenses (PALs). The Correction of Myopia Evaluation Trial (COMET) study is the largest double randomized, double masked clinical trial that evaluates the effect of PALs versus SVLs on the progression of myopia in children. Although clinically insignificant, the study revealed decreased mean increase of myopia in children treated with PALs, compared to children with SVLs [13, 19].

A similar study conducted by Hasebe et al. investigated the effects of PALs versus SVLs on slowing the progression of myopia using a crossover design, which switches the spectacle type at the half of the study. At the end of this 3-year study period, progression was less in the group wearing PALs first than the group with SVLs first. The study concludes that early intervention with PALs is more effective that SVLs in controlling myopia, slowing progression and halting axial elongation of the eye [20]. Several other statistically significant, but clinically insignificant, studies have explored the use of PALs compared to SVLs for slowing the progression of myopia [21–23]. With more large population and long duration studies, the studies can achieve statistical and clinical significance in preventing myopia progression and axial elongation.

Myovision lenses appear similar to SVLs, but they are a newer design of spectacles that correct central and side vision that are experimented on many myopic Asian pediatric populations. The mechanism of these spectacles is to reduce the peripheral hyperopia and prevent myopia progression. These lenses resemble SVLs in appearance, are comfortable to wear and easy to adapt to the young population [24]. Similar studies with MyoVision lenses on Japanese children, which reveal an insignificant difference between the effect of MyoVision lenses and SVL wearers on spherical equivalent refraction and axial elongation of the eye [25].

At this early stage of exploration, the efficacy of MyoVision lenses are not yet fully understood or proven. With additional studies that can reduce peripheral hyperopic defocus more effectively, there is more potential for reduction of myopia progression and axial elongation.

2.1.2 Contact lens correction

Majority of the myopic population advocate for contact lenses are from the adult population, as it produces cosmetic benefits in addition to functional improvement of the vision and their quality of life. However, contact lenses, such as rigid gas permeable contact lens, have also been utilized in the pediatric population to retard myopia progression and decrease axial elongation.

Rigid gas permeable contact lenses have been shown to retard myopia progression in studies such as, The Contact Lens and Myopia Progression (CLAMP), which explored the progression of myopia in rigid gas permeable contact lens wearers versus soft lens controls. The CLAMP study reported that in 2 years the myopia progression was less in rigid gas permeable wearers ($-1.56 \pm 0.95D$) than in soft contact lens wearers ($-2.19 \pm 0.89D$) [11, 26]. Numerous other studies have demonstrated that the provisional decrease in myopia progression in rigid gas permeable contact lens wearers in comparison to other treatment groups, was a consequence of flattening of the cornea, and not the axial length of the eye [26–28].

Soft bifocal contact lens has demonstrated slowing of myopia progression by reducing the accommodation effort and halting axial elongation [29]. These lenses are designed with power for distance in the center and additional power in the periphery, or inversely, which corrects central myopia and reduces relative peripheral hyperopia. A study conducted by Walline et al. compared the effects of soft multifocal contact lenses with single vision lenses, and reported that the average myopic progression at 2 years was 0.41 ± 0.03D for the single-vision contact lens wearers and 0.29 ± 0.03D for the soft multifocal contact lens wearers [29]. While the study produced statistically significant results, it was clinically insignificant.

Using a contralateral eye study design, Anstice et al. demonstrated that the eye wearing soft bifocal contact lens have a slower axial elongation in comparison to the eye wearing soft single vision contact lens. However, this was not clinically significant [30].

There is much potential for soft bifocal contact lenses to reduce myopic progression and axial elongation, which can be achieved with future large-scale studies that explore the mechanism of myopic control through reduced accommodation effort and studies that compare the effectiveness of soft bifocal contact lens with other modes of optical control of myopia.

Orthokeratology is a technique used in the reduction of myopia by flattening the cornea by the rigid orthokeratology contact lenses. The pattern of lens wear in this correction technique allows for the correction of myopia for short periods of time. The lenses are worn overnight to temporarily alter the corneal shape by corneal thinning, are removed during the day when the visual acuity would be improved temporarily [31]. The Berkeley Orthokeratology study demonstrated a significantly greater reduction of myopia in orthokeratology contact lens wearers, in comparison to a control group. However, the study was not clinically significant [9, 32].

The Longitudinal Orthokeratology Research in Children study was explored the effects of Orthokeratology contact lenses worn for 2 years on children in Hong Kong. At the study end, the there was a significant difference in the axial length between the lens wearers and the control group, 0.29 and 0.54 mm, respectively. The study was not clinically significant, represents the need for large scale studies to achieve clinical and statistical significance [31, 33].

With additional studies that can reduce peripheral hyperopic defocus more effectively, there is more potential for reduction of myopia progression and axial elongation.

2.2 Pharmacological management

2.2.1 Atropine

Atropine is a non-selective muscarinic antagonist that has been the most effective in slowing the progression of myopia. One theory for the mechanism of atropine is the role of scleral remodeling in myopia and axial elongation. The expression of the muscarinic receptors (mAChRs) results in the proliferation of fibroblasts in the scleral collagenous matrix, which promotes scleral remodeling and ultimately axial elongation [34]. Some axial elongation induced morphological scleral changes include lamellar arrangement of collagen fibers in myopic eyes rather than the tight interwoven collagen fibers in emmetropic eyes, the reduction in fibril diameter, a dispersed range of fibril diameters, and an increased number of abnormal fibrils represent are representations [35, 36]. It is theorized that atropine receptor blockage interrupts scleral fibroblast proliferation and consequential axial elongation of the eye. Although the mechanism of atropine remains obscure, there are several working theories on the action and effect of this drug on myopia progression and axial elongation.

The Atropine in the Treatment of Myopia (ATOM) study was conducted from 1999 to 2004, which explored the effect of atropine 1% instilled nightly in children in Singapore for 2 years. The study contained two phases: a 2-year treatment phase and a 1-year washout phase. At the end of the 2-year study period, there was a

77% reduction in myopia progression with an unaltered axial length, compared to the control [37, 38]. The study was originally conducted in Asia but was adopted by other countries due to its encouraging results [39–43]. Following a successful 2-year treatment phase, the patients displayed rebound phenomenon in the 1-year washout phase. During this phase, there was an increase in both refractive error and axial length [37, 38]. The instillation of topical atropine was generally tolerated with some short- and long-term side effects. Short-term side effects are red eyes, photophobia, dilatation, increased intraocular pressure and glaucoma, and long-term side effects include retinal vascular diseases and cataract formation [37, 38]. The ATOM study was proved highly effective in reducing the rate of axial elongation and myopia progression, but was associated with such expected side effects.

Following the ATOM1 study was a 5-year clinical trial, which investigates low-dose atropine on reducing the progression of myopia, and subsequently decreasing the side effects. ATOM2 participants were randomly assigned to receive 0.5, 0.1 or 0.01% concentration of atropine for 24 months, followed by a 1-year washout phase. The results of ATOM2 study reveals that 0.01% is a viable concentration for reducing myopia progression and increasing the safety profile [44, 45].

While both ATOM and ATOM2 studies display efficacy in reducing myopia progression, both studies reveal a dose-dependent rebound phenomenon during the washout period. More recently, The Low-Concentration Atropine for Myopia Progression (LAMP) study was conducted to evaluate the efficacy and safety of low concentrations of atropine eye drops including 0.05, 0.025 and 0.01% compared to a placebo. The LAMP study revealed that all three low concentrations of atropine reduce myopia without a discernable adverse effect on the visual quality of life, and 0.05% was the most effective in controlling the spherical equivalent progression and the axial elongation over the 1-year study period [46]. Numerous studies have compared the effect of atropine to other optical strategies, such as single vision lenses, multifocal lenses, rigid gas permeable contact lenses, and orthokeratology [47–49].

Combination studies have explored the effects of atropine and an optical correction for greater myopia control. Shih et al. demonstrated that multifocal lens wearers treated with 0.5% atropine have a greater reduction of axial elongation and myopia progression, compared to placebo group [50]. Atropine eye drops for the treatment of myopia control has gained wide popularity in Asian countries, and more recently it has been adopted by the Western countries as well. With further investigation and modification to the treatment regimen that evades rebound phenomenon, atropine has the potential to be the conventional treatment of myopia.

2.2.2 Pirenzepine

Pirenzepine is a selective M1 muscarinic receptor antagonist with a similar mechanism as atropine in halting myopia progression and axial elongation. A study conducted by Siatkowski et al. developed a 2% pirenzepine gel that displayed great efficacy in reduction of refractive error compared to the placebo group. Additionally, the average axial length increase at 1 year was 0.19 mm for patients in pirenzepine treatment group compared to 0.23 mm for those in the placebo group. While the results are statistically significant, they are clinically insignificant [51]. The adverse events in patients treated with pirenzepine were mild to moderately severe and included mydriasis, erythema of eyelids and ocular itching [9, 51, 52]. Overall, the study displayed good safety and efficacy for use in myopia control. Future studies are warranted to compare the efficacy and safety of pirenzepine and atropine in slowing the progression of myopia and axial elongation. Atropine eye drops for the treatment of myopia control has gained wide popularity in Asian countries, and more recently it has been adopted by the Western countries as well. With further investigation and modification to the treatment regimen that evades rebound phenomenon, atropine has the potential to be the conventional treatment of myopia.

2.2.3 Anti-hypoxic drugs

Anti-hypoxic drugs such as salidroside and formononetin have shown anti-hypoxic effects to treat scleral hypoxia in myopia [53, 54]. Scleral hypoxia, which is induced by Hypoxia-Inducible Factor-1α (HIF-1), triggers a signaling cascade for myofibroblast trans-differentiation leading to scleral extracellular collagenous matrix remodeling in progressing myopia [55]. Formononetin is known decrease HIF-1α, vascular endothelial growth factor (VEGF) and prolyl hydroxylase domain-2 (PHD-2), which are protective in hypoxia-induced retinal neovascularization [54]. Salidroside is protective against for hypoxia-induced cardiac apoptosis and pulmonary hypertension [56, 57].

In animal models with experimentally induced myopia, anti-hypoxic drugs down-regulated HIF-1α expression and the phosphorylation levels of eIF2α and mTOR to inhibit the development of form deprivation myopia, without affecting the normal ocular growth in guinea pigs [55]. Due to encouraging results in animal models, the use of anti-hypoxic drugs shows great potential for treatment of myopia in human eyes.

2.3 Surgical management

Surgeons have recently advocated for surgical intervention to halt the progression of myopia, axial elongation and weakening of the posterior sclera. Macular buckle surgery or posterior reinforcement (PSR) surgery is proven to be effective in reinforcing the weakened posterior sclera. A scleral buckle is used to apply direct mechanical force onto the posterior pole, which slows the axial elongation. Shen et al. documented significantly higher Best-Corrected Visual Acuity (BCVA) and lower refractive error in the group who underwent macular buckle surgery compared to the control group [58]. Additionally, patients who underwent PSR surgery have a shorter mean axial length and lower mean refractive error than the control group [59, 60].

Macular buckling surgery has also been used myopic macular hole with retinal detachment and posterior staphyloma, which displayed high reattachment rates and improved visual acuity [61, 62]. Recent studies have experimented with different buckle materials, shapes, techniques and other modifications for the best correction of myopia and its complications [63–65]. With more advanced techniques and modifications, the surgical technique can be utilized as conventional treatment of myopia to reduce myopia progression and axial elongation.

3. Conclusion

The global prevalence of myopia is in an increasing trend, with estimates of myopia and high myopia affecting nearly 5 billion and 1 billion people, respectively, in 2050 [1]. As a major public health concern, it is essential to develop interventions that sufficiently delay or stop the progression of myopia. Of the above discussed treatments, all have shown to reduce the progression of myopia, but atropine has been the most popular and effective in reducing progression and axial elongation. Despite the expected side effects, its rebound phenomenon and its obscure mechanism, atropine has achieved global popularity. With changes in lifestyle, health education, government and other health systems, the importance and acceptance of myopia control will significantly diminish number of people affected. Additionally, the implementation of a conventional, safe and effective intervention for myopia control will significantly reduce the personal, societal and economic burden, and decrease the disease progression and the risk of future myopia-induced ocular complications.

Conflict of interest

There are no financial conflicts of interest.

Author details

Sangeethabalasri Pugazhendhi[1], Balamurali Ambati[2] and Allan A. Hunter[3]*

1 PSG Institute of Medical Sciences and Research, India

2 Pacific ClearVision Institute, Oregon, USA

3 Oregon Eye Consultants, Eugene, Oregon, USA

*Address all correspondence to: hunter.allan.a@gmail.com

IntechOpen

© 2019 The Author(s). Licensee IntechOpen. This chapter is distributed under the terms of the Creative Commons Attribution License (http://creativecommons.org/licenses/by/3.0), which permits unrestricted use, distribution, and reproduction in any medium, provided the original work is properly cited.

References

[1] Holden BA et al. Global prevalence of myopia and high myopia and temporal trends from 2000 through 2050. Ophthalmology. 2016;**123**(5):1036-1042

[2] Morgan IG et al. The epidemics of myopia: Aetiology and prevention. Progress in Retinal and Eye Research. 2018;**62**:134-149

[3] Cook RC, Glasscock RE. Refractive and ocular findings in the newborn. American Journal of Ophthalmology. 1951;**34**(10):1407-1413

[4] Goldschmidt E. Refraction in the newborn. Acta Ophthalmologica. 1969;**47**(3):570-578

[5] Wallman J, Winawer J. Homeostasis of eye growth and the question of myopia. Neuron. 2004;**43**(4):447-468

[6] Gordon RA, Donzis PB. Refractive development of the human eye. Archives of Ophthalmology. 1985;**103**(6):785-789

[7] Ehrlich DL et al. Infant emmetropization: Longitudinal changes in refraction components from nine to twenty months of age. Optometry and Vision Science. 1997;**74**(10):822-843

[8] Smith MJ, Walline JJ. Controlling myopia progression in children and adolescents. Adolescent Health, Medicine and Therapeutics. 2015;**6**:133-140

[9] Saw SM et al. Myopia: Attempts to arrest progression. The British Journal of Ophthalmology. 2002;**86**(11):1306-1311

[10] Myrowitz EH. Juvenile myopia progression, risk factors and interventions. Saudi journal of ophthalmology. 2012;**26**(3):293-297

[11] Walline JJ. Myopia control: A review. Eye Contact Lens. 2016;**42**(1):3-8

[12] Smith EL 3rd. Spectacle lenses and emmetropization: The role of optical defocus in regulating ocular development. Optometry and Vision Science. 1998;**75**(6):388-398

[13] Gwiazda J. Treatment options for myopia. Optometry and Vision Science: Official Publication of the American Academy of Optometry. 2009;**86**(6):624-628

[14] Hung LF, Crawford ML, Smith EL. Spectacle lenses alter eye growth and the refractive status of young monkeys. Nature Medicine. 1995;**1**(8):761-765

[15] Hung GK, Ciuffreda KJ. Quantitative analysis of the effect of near lens addition on accommodation and myopigenesis. Current Eye Research. 2000;**20**(4):293-312

[16] Curtin BJ, Jampol LM. The myopias: Basic science and clinical management. Harper & Row, 1985;**6**(2):132

[17] Chung K, Mohidin N, O'Leary DJ. Undercorrection of myopia enhances rather than inhibits myopia progression. Vision Research. 2002;**42**(22):2555-2559

[18] Adler D, Millodot M. The possible effect of undercorrection on myopic progression in children. Clinical & Experimental Optometry. 2006;**89**(5):315-321

[19] Gwiazda J et al. Progressive-addition lenses versus single-vision lenses for slowing progression of myopia in children with high accommodative lag and near esophoria. Investigative Ophthalmology & Visual Science. 2011;**52**(5):2749-2757

[20] Hasebe S et al. Effect of progressive addition lenses on myopia progression in Japanese children: A prospective, randomized, double-masked, crossover trial. Investigative Ophthalmology & Visual Science. 2008;**49**(7):2781-2789

[21] Cheng D et al. Randomized trial of effect of bifocal and prismatic bifocal spectacles on myopic progression: Two-year results. Archives of Ophthalmology. 2010;**128**(1):12-19

[22] Fulk GW, Cyert LA, Parker DE. A randomized clinical trial of bifocal glasses for myopic children with esophoria: Results after 54 months. Optometry. 2002;**73**(8):470-476

[23] Yang Z et al. The effectiveness of progressive addition lenses on the progression of myopia in Chinese children. Ophthalmic & Physiological Optics. 2009;**29**(1):41-48

[24] Sankaridurg P et al. Spectacle lenses designed to reduce progression of myopia: 12-month results. Optometry and Vision Science: Official Publication of the American Academy of Optometry. 2010;**87**(9):631-641

[25] Kanda H et al. Effect of spectacle lenses designed to reduce relative peripheral hyperopia on myopia progression in Japanese children: A 2-year multicenter randomized controlled trial. Japanese Journal of Ophthalmology. 2018;**62**(5):537-543

[26] Walline JJ et al. The contact lens and myopia progression (CLAMP) study: Design and baseline data. Optometry and Vision Science. 2001;**78**(4):223-233

[27] Grosvenor T et al. Rigid gas-permeable contact lenses for myopia control: Effects of discontinuation of lens wear. Optometry and Vision Science. 1991;**68**(5):385-389

[28] Khoo CY, Chong J, Rajan U. A 3-year study on the effect of RGP contact lenses on myopic children. Singapore Medical Journal. 1999;**40**(4):230-237

[29] Walline JJ et al. Multifocal contact lens myopia control. Optometry and Vision Science. 2013;**90**(11):1207-1214

[30] Anstice NS, Phillips JR. Effect of dual-focus soft contact lens wear on axial myopia progression in children. Ophthalmology. 2011;**118**(6):1152-1161

[31] Leo SW, Young TL. An evidence-based update on myopia and interventions to retard its progression. Journal of AAPOS. 2011;**15**(2):181-189

[32] Polse KA et al. The berkeley orthokeratology study, Part II: Efficacy and duration. American Journal of Optometry and Physiological Optics. 1983;**60**(3):187-198

[33] Cho P, Cheung SW, Edwards M. The longitudinal orthokeratology research in children (LORIC) in Hong Kong: A pilot study on refractive changes and myopic control. Current Eye Research. 2005;**30**(1):71-80

[34] Barathi VA, Weon SR, Beuerman RW. Expression of muscarinic receptors in human and mouse sclera and their role in the regulation of scleral fibroblasts proliferation. Molecular Vision. 2009;**15**:1277-1293

[35] Curtin BJ, Iwamoto T, Renaldo DP. Normal and staphylomatous sclera of high myopia. An electron microscopic study. Archives of Ophthalmology. 1979;**97**(5):912-915

[36] McBrien NA, Gentle A. Role of the sclera in the development and pathological complications of myopia. Progress in Retinal and Eye Research. 2003;**22**(3):307-338

[37] Lee CY et al. Effects of topical atropine on intraocular pressure and myopia progression: A prospective comparative study. BMC Ophthalmology. 2016;**16**:114

[38] Chua WH et al. Atropine for the treatment of childhood myopia. Ophthalmology. 2006;**113**(12):2285-2291

[39] Brodstein RS et al. The treatment of myopia with atropine and bifocals. A long-term prospective study. Ophthalmology. 1984;**91**(11):1373-1379

[40] Li SM et al. Atropine slows myopia progression more in Asian than white children by meta-analysis. Optometry and Vision Science. 2014;**91**(3):342-350

[41] Clark TY, Clark RA. Atropine 0.01% eyedrops significantly reduce the progression of childhood myopia. Journal of Ocular Pharmacology and Therapeutics. 2015;**31**(9):541-545

[42] Kothari M, Rathod V. Efficacy of 1% atropine eye drops in retarding progressive axial myopia in Indian eyes. Indian Journal of Ophthalmology. 2017;**65**(11):1178-1181

[43] Polling JR et al. Effectiveness study of atropine for progressive myopia in Europeans. Eye (London, England). 2016;**30**(7):998-1004

[44] Chia A et al. Atropine for the treatment of childhood myopia: Safety and efficacy of 0.5%, 0.1%, and 0.01% doses (Atropine for the treatment of myopia 2). Ophthalmology. 2012;**119**(2):347-354

[45] Chia A, Lu QS, Tan D. Five-year clinical trial on atropine for the treatment of myopia 2: Myopia control with atropine 0.01% eyedrops. Ophthalmology. 2016;**123**(2):391-399

[46] Yam JC et al. Low-Concentration Atropine for Myopia Progression (LAMP) Study: A randomized, double-blinded, placebo-controlled trial of 0.05%, 0.025%, and 0.01% atropine eye drops in myopia control. Ophthalmology. 2019;**126**(1):113-124

[47] Hsiao CK et al. Design and statistical analysis for the myopia intervention trial in Taiwan. In: Myopia Updates II. Tokyo: Springer Japan; 2000

[48] Lin H-J et al. Overnight orthokeratology is comparable with atropine in controlling myopia. BMC Ophthalmology. 2014;**14**(1):40

[49] Wan L, Wei CC, Chen CS, et al. The Synergistic effects of orthokeratology and atropine in slowing the progression of myopia. Journal of Clinical Medicine. 2018;**7**(9):259

[50] Shih YF et al. An intervention trial on efficacy of atropine and multi-focal glasses in controlling myopic progression. Acta Ophthalmologica Scandinavica. 2001;**79**(3):233-236

[51] Siatkowski RM et al. Safety and efficacy of 2% pirenzepine ophthalmic gel in children with myopia: A 1-year, multicenter, double-masked, placebo-controlled parallel study. Archives of Ophthalmology. 2004;**122**(11):1667-1674

[52] Truong HT et al. Pirenzepine affects scleral metabolic changes in myopia through a non-toxic mechanism. Experimental Eye Research. 2002;**74**(1):103-111

[53] Xu ZW et al. SILAC-based proteomic analysis reveals that salidroside antagonizes cobalt chloride-induced hypoxic effects by restoring the tricarboxylic acid cycle in cardiomyocytes. Journal of Proteomics. 2016;**130**:211-220

[54] Wu J et al. Formononetin, an active compound of Astragalus membranaceus (Fisch) Bunge, inhibits hypoxia-induced retinal neovascularization via the HIF-1alpha/VEGF signaling pathway. Drug Design, Development and Therapy. 2016;**10**:3071-3081

[55] Wu H et al. Scleral hypoxia is a target for myopia control. Proceedings of the National Academy of Sciences of the United States of America. 2018;**115**(30):E7091-e7100

[56] Lai MC et al. Protective effect of salidroside on cardiac apoptosis in mice with chronic intermittent hypoxia. International Journal of Cardiologyl. 2014;**174**(3):565-573

[57] Huang X et al. Salidroside attenuates chronic hypoxia-induced pulmonary hypertension via adenosine A2a receptor related mitochondria-dependent apoptosis pathway. Journal of Molecular and Cellular Cardiology. 2015;**82**:153-166

[58] Shen ZM et al. Posterior scleral reinforcement combined with patching therapy for pre-school children with unilateral high myopia. Graefe's Archive for Clinical and Experimental Ophthalmology. 2015;**253**(8):1391-1395

[59] Li X-J et al. Posterior scleral reinforcement for the treatment of pathological myopia. International journal of ophthalmology. 2016;**9**(4):580-584

[60] Liu XD, Lu JH, Chu RY. Long-term studies on clinical therapeutic efficiency of posterior scleral reinforcement surgery. Zhonghua Yan Ke Za Zhi. 2011;**47**(6):527-530

[61] Theodossiadis GP, Theodossiadis PG. The macular buckling procedure in the treatment of retinal detachment in highly myopic eyes with macular hole and posterior staphyloma: Mean follow-up of 15 years. Retina. 2005;**25**(3):285-289

[62] Sasoh M et al. Macular buckling for retinal detachment due to macular hole in highly myopic eyes with posterior staphyloma. Retina. 2000;**20**(5):445-449

[63] Parolini B et al. Indications and results of a new l-shaped macular buckle to support a posterior staphyloma in high myopia. Retina. 2015;**35**(12):2469-2482

[64] Devin F et al. T-shaped scleral buckle for macular detachments in high myopes. Retina. 2011;**31**(1):177-180

[65] Stirpe M et al. A new adjustable macular buckle designed for highly myopic eyes. Retina, 2012;**32**(7):1424-1427

Chapter 8

Surgical Correction of Myopia

Maja Bohac, Maja Pauk Gulic, Alma Biscevic and Ivan Gabric

Abstract

Myopia is the most prevalent refractive error in the world and its incidence is increasing. Together with conservative methods of treatment, various surgical methods have been proposed. Corneal refractive surgery is probably the most accepted one. Laser in situ keratomileusis (LASIK), photorefractive keratectomy (PRK), and small incision lenticule extraction (SMILE) are suitable for treatment of myopia up to −8.00 D in the younger age group. For patients not suitable for corneal refractive surgery, lens-based procedures are available. Phakic intraocular lenses are suitable for patients younger than 45 years of age with high myopia or some other contraindications for corneal refractive surgery. For older patients, refractive lens exchange (RLE) with implantation of multifocal or monofocal intraocular lenses is gaining popularity.

Keywords: myopia, LASIK, PRK, SMILE, phakic intraocular lenses, refractive lens exchange

1. Introduction

Myopia is a common refractive error in the population. It is defined as an optical aberration in which parallel light rays from a distant image are getting focused on a point anterior to the retina. Hereditary and environmental factors both play an important role in the development of myopia. Myopia typically appears between the age of 6 and 12, and the mean rate of progression is considered to be approximately 0.50 D per year, based on studies of mostly Caucasian children. One of the studies showed that progression of myopia can vary by ethnicity, as well as by age of the child. For instance, in ethnic Chinese children, the progression rate is higher [1].

A recent report in *Nature*, entitled "The Myopia Boom," demonstrated, and it is now widely accepted, that there is an epidemic of myopia in the developed countries of East and Southeast Asia, paralleled by an epidemic of high myopia [2]. Recent meta-analyses have suggested that close to half of the world's population may be myopic by 2050, with as much as 10% highly myopic [3]. Correction of refractive error can be achieved conservatively with glasses or contact lenses which is the treatment of choice in the childhood. However, despite the long-standing use of glasses and contact lenses, there are some disadvantages in both forms of optical correction. Increased light scatter, image magnification/minification, discomfort, and inconvenience are some of the issues with glasses, while contact lenses may irritate the ocular surface with increased risk of corneal scratches and infections. After the age of 21, various surgical treatments can be considered. The best surgical option depends on the amount of refractive error and the patient's cornea, lens, and age. Available options include various laser vision corrections which are aimed on the cornea, implantation of phakic intraocular lenses (pIOLs), and refractive lens exchange (RLE) with implantation of multifocal and monofocal intraocular lenses (IOLs). It is important to perform a detailed examination of each patient and assess their needs, wishes, and expectations. Doctors need to explain in as much detail as possible what the expected results and risk would be with for the selected surgical method.

2. Corneal refractive surgery

Procedures which involve altering the shape of the cornea with excimer laser are collectively referred to as keratorefractive surgery, refractive keratoplasty, laser vision correction, or refractive corneal surgery.

2.1 Photorefractive keratectomy

Photorefractive keratectomy (PRK) was the first excimer laser technique for the treatment of refractive errors. Seiler performed the first corneal ablation in a live patient in 1985, and McDonald treated the first human sighted eye in 1985 after extensive preclinical investigation [4]. The PRK procedure involves removal of the central corneal epithelium, most commonly performed mechanically (brush, crescent knife, or alcohol) or with excimer laser when it is referred as transepithelial PRK (T-PRK). The denuded anterior stroma is then reshaped by the excimer laser, with either central corneal flattening, steepening, or a torical pattern when treating myopia, hyperopia, or astigmatism, respectively. Due to significant postoperative pain, relatively slow visual recovery, epithelial defects due to irregular healing, and haze development, especially when treating high myopia [5, 6], different techniques of epithelial removal were introduced over time to solve these complications [7]. Recently the role of surface ablations has been reevaluated due to raised issues of potential flap complications, risk of iatrogenic corneal ectasia, and inability to treat thin corneas with laser in situ keratomileusis (LASIK) [8]. With surface ablation techniques, there is no flap involved, and more cornea tissue is preserved, and by some it is still considered the overall safest procedure for treatment of low to moderate myopia [9]. It is performed, especially in corneas with superficial scarring, epithelial dystrophies, or recurrent erosions, in thin corneas, after penetrating keratoplasty and for keratorefractive retreatments. The introduction of mitomycin C and modern surface ablation techniques has also increased the range of treatment and lowered the risk of haze and regression after PRK [10]. Therefore today surface ablation includes several sub-techniques such as epithelial LASIK (epi-LASIK), laser-assisted subepithelial keratectomy (LASEK), and T-PRK [11].

2.2 Laser in situ keratomileusis

The term LASIK was first used in 1990 by Pallikaris [4]. The procedure is performed in two steps. The first step involves the formation of a front corneal flap and the lifting of the flap for the purpose of exposing the corneal stroma. The hinged flap consists of the corneal epithelium, the Bowman membrane, and superficial stroma. The second step is the application of the excimer laser on the stromal bed. Once the ablation with the excimer laser is finished, the flap is returned into its original position.

LASIK has now become the most common elective surgical procedure in the world, presumably because it is almost painless with fast visual recovery, as compared to PRK [4]. Nowadays, there are two techniques available for the formation of the flap—mechanical microkeratomes and femtosecond lasers. The use of femtosecond laser-assisted laser in situ keratomileusis (FsLASIK) offers greater precision in flap creation leading to better morphological stability of the flap compared to earlier bladed microkeratome keratomileusis. However, changes in the biomechanical strength of the cornea, induction of higher-order aberrations, and flap-related complications can still occur [12]. LASIK reduces the tensile strength of the stroma by about 35% when the ablation takes place between 10 and 30% of the stromal depth [13]. Regarding the available data, and our experience, there is no significant difference in shorter-term refractive stability and induction of high-order aberrations between T-PRK and LASIK (**Figures 1** and **2** and **Table 1**). However, when higher refractive errors are treated, surface ablations pose more risk for haze development and regression [14].

2.3 Small incision lenticule extraction

The femtosecond laser corneal procedure known as small incision lenticule extraction (SMILE) was originally described by Sekundo et al. and became clinically

	preop	1 week postop	1 month postop	3 month postop	6 month postop
LASIK	-4,26	-0,19	-0,12	-0,2	-0,06
PRK	-4,22	-0,27	-0,25	-0,33	-0,25

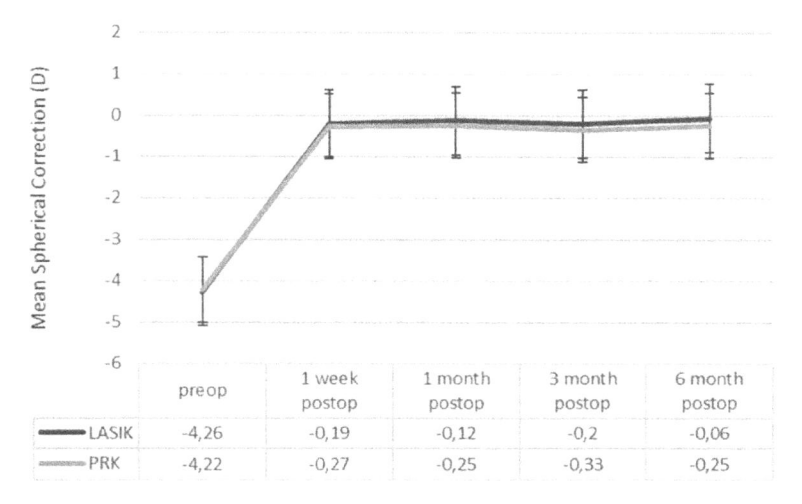

Figure 1.
Comparison of change in spherical correction over time between T-PRK and LASIK.

	preop	1 week postop	1 month postop	3 month postop	6 month postop
LASIK	-0,75	-0,11	-0,12	-0,17	-0,06
PRK	-0,79	-0,57	-0,48	-0,3	-0,18

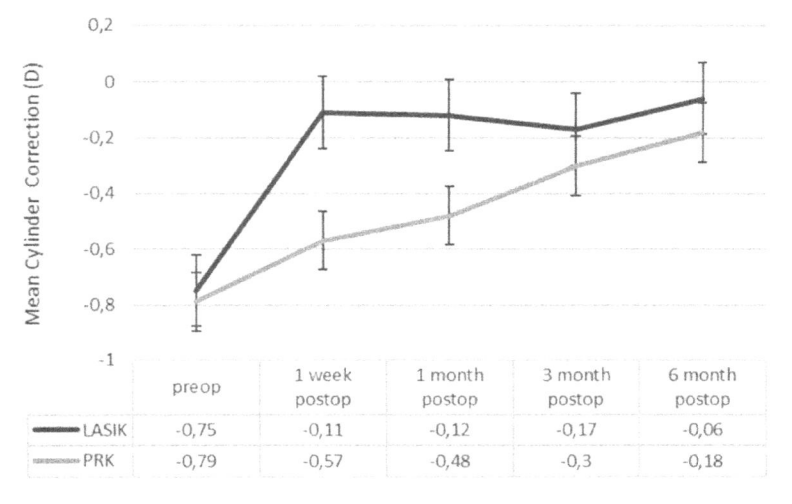

Figure 2.
Comparison of change in astigmatism correction over time between T-PRK and LASIK.

HIGH ORDER ABERRATIONS AT 5mm PUPIL

	T-PRK			LASIK		
	PreOp	3 month postop	6 month postop	PreOp	3 month postop	6 month postop
COMA (μm)	0,12±0,07	0,15±0,09	0,13±0,1	0,9±0,07	0,13±0,09	0,09±0,07
TREFOIL (μm)	0,08±0,05	0,14±0,08	0,10±0,06	0,09±0,05	0,10±0,05	0,08±0,08
SA (μm)	-0,01±0,05	-0,01±0,07	-0,01±0,05	0,1±0,09	0,01±0,05	0,02±0,03

Table 1.
Comparison of change in high-order aberrations over time between T-PRK and LASIK.

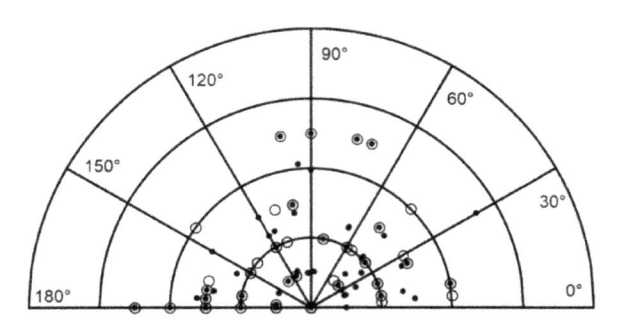

Figure 3.
Polar diagram showing target and surgically induced astigmatic values for the SMILE group. The concentric semicircles reduce in 0.50 D steps from −2.00 DC (outermost semicircle) toward zero (central point) in 0.50 DC steps. From right to left, the 0 to 90 to 180° axes are shown in 30° steps. The target and surgically induced astigmatism data points are shown as empty circles and filled dots, respectively.

available in 2011 [15]. The procedure does not require the creation of a flap: two precise intrastromal planar sections are created using a single femtosecond laser to form an intrastromal lenticule. The intrastromal lenticule is dissected from the pocket, grasped with a forceps, and manually extracted through a small incision. The incision is placed at the superior temporal/nasal quadrant, usually angled at 70°, and 2–5 mm in length. The removal of the intrastromal lenticule alters the shape of the cornea, thereby correcting myopia and astigmatism. Since Bowman's layer remains intact, the procedure offers greater biomechanical stability, especially in the treatment of higher levels of myopia [15]. The flapless property of SMILE obviates the risks associated with LASIK including adverse events at flap creation and dislocation [16].

The tensile strength of the cornea may reduce by 55% after a SMILE procedure when the lenticule is formed and extracted from the anterior half of the stroma. Loss of tensile strength is less profound when the lenticule is extracted from deeper regions of the stroma. Thus, the exact change in the biomechanical properties of the cornea will depend on the amount of ablation and the location where the lenticule is formed [13].

Regarding the available data, and our experience, LASIK and SMILE are comparable procedures in terms of visual quality and reduction of myopia; however, in treating astigmatism LASIK still offers better precision (**Figures 3 and 4**).

2.4 Indications and preoperative preparation for refractive surgery

A detailed review of the patient's condition before surgery and informing the patient about the results, benefits, and disadvantages of the procedure are the most important steps for a successful outcome of refractive surgery [17].

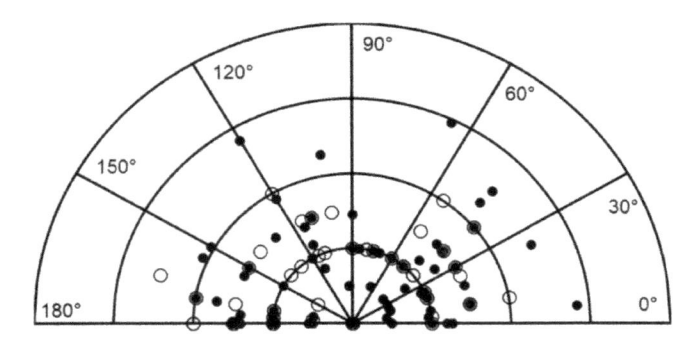

Figure 4.
Polar diagram showing target and surgically induced astigmatic values for the FsLASIK group. The concentric semicircles reduce in 0.50 D steps from −2.00 DC (outermost semicircle) toward zero (central point) in 0.50 DC steps. From right to left, the 0 to 90 to 180° axes are shown in 30° steps. The target and surgically induced astigmatism data points are shown as empty circles and filled dots, respectively.

The examination should include detailed medical history (systemic status, medications intake, allergies, ocular status, information about previous ocular surgeries—especially in the case of refractive lens exchange—and information about contact lens wear) and reasons/motivations for refractive surgery to identify patients with unrealistic expectations [18, 19]. It is important for patients to understand that refractive surgery primarily serves to reduce spectacle dependence and contact lens use, and it is not meant to completely remove all optical aids in all situations, for an indefinite time period.

Patients should discontinue contact lens use before the examination (for soft contact lenses, at least a week prior to the examination, and for rigid gas permeable contact lenses, at least 2–3 weeks prior) since corneal topography and biometry measurement can be severely affected by the corneal changes induced by contact lens wear. In the case of corneal warpage syndrome (corneal irregularities caused by contact lenses), contact lenses should be discontinued for at least 4–6 weeks [20].

The preoperative evaluation must include monocular manifest refraction, cycloplegic refraction, uncorrected distance visual acuity (UDVA), corrected distance visual acuity (CDVA), pupillometry, tonometry, anterior chamber depth (ACD) measurement, corneal topography/tomography, pachymetry, aberrometry, tear film quality and quantity, determining the dominant eye, ocular motility, and a fundus examination [18, 21]. Cycloplegic refraction is recommended to exclude the accommodation effect, while in patients in/or close to presbyopia age near visual acuity should be checked also. It is mandatory to check the patient's refractive stability during the time, which can most often be obtained by inspecting the patient's eyeglasses or by reviewing the previous ophthalmological documentation [21].

Contraindications for refractive surgery may relate to systemic or ocular disorders. Absolute systemic contraindications are poorly controlled systemic immune diseases (e.g., rheumatoid arthritis, systemic lupus erythematosus, polyarteritis nodosa), as well as poorly controlled diabetes and AIDS. Such patients have a higher risk of complications associated with prolonged inflammation or corneal healing after refractive surgery [18, 22–24]. Surgical procedures are not recommended during pregnancy and lactation [25].

Ocular absolute contraindications are considered to be poorly controlled or untreated eye inflammation (blepharitis, dry eye syndrome, atopy/allergy), poorly controlled glaucoma, clinically significant lens opacities, Stevens-Johnson syndrome, ocular pemphigoid, and chemical burns of the eye surface [26, 27]. Instability of refraction (i.e., a change greater than 0.50 D within a year) is considered as an absolute contraindication, as well as insufficient corneal thickness or corneal irregularities suspicious for keratoconus [21, 26, 28, 29]. Precautions are also needed in patients with certain systemic therapies (isotretinoin, amiodarone, sumatriptan, colchicine) [23, 24, 30]. Caution is also required in functional monocular patients and in patients with well-controlled glaucoma. Other relative contraindications are history of uveitis, herpes simplex, and varicella zoster keratitis. In patients with epithelial basal membrane degeneration, LASIK is not recommended, but PRK is the procedure to consider [21, 31].

2.5 Limitations and complications of corneal refractive surgery

Complications of corneal refractive surgery are considered rare. They can be divided in intraoperative and postoperative complications (which can be early or delayed).

Regarding the intraoperative complications, they are mainly correlated with corneal flap creation or excimer laser ablation. During the era of microkeratome, flap-related complications were encountered more often and fell within 3%; with the introduction of femtosecond lasers, they were almost nullified; however, some complications specific to femtosecond lasers appeared [32].

Flap-related complications include free or partial flap creation, incomplete and irregular flap creation, thin and perforated flaps, and corneal perforation. Those complications were mostly related to corneal anatomy (flat <41.00 D or steep >46.00 D corneas, small corneal diameter), inadequate suction, mechanical failure—a defect in the dissection blade or motor unit—and surgeon experience. Penetration into the anterior chamber is extremely rare and may occur during lamellar dissection or excimer laser photoablation usually on extremely thin corneas with old scars [33].

Femtosecond-related complications are closely correlated with cavitation bubbles and formation of the flap. They are presented in the form of confluent cavitation bubbles in the corneal lamellae or anterior chamber which can interfere with excimer laser systems and vertical gas breakthrough which is presented in the forms of incomplete buttonholes or difficulties in dissecting the flap due to tissue bridges [34]. Temporary hypersensitivity to light and rainbow glare are complications exclusively related to energy and pattern of femtosecond lasers characterized with normal visual acuity and photophobia without inflammation or light dispersion in low light conditions [35].

Laser-related complications include decentration of excimer laser ablation, irregular astigmatism, and formation of central islands. Those complications are clinically characterized by poor uncorrected and corrected distance visual acuity complaints of glare, "ghosting" around images and haloes, and refractive astigmatism in the axis of decentration [33].

Early postoperative complications include flap striae, diffuse lamellar keratitis, central toxic keratopathy, pressure-induced steroid keratitis, infectious keratitis, and epithelial ingrowth.

Flap striae are caused by misalignment of the flap; peripheral striae usually are asymptomatic; however, central location of the striae is associated with loss in corrected distance visual acuity and night vision disturbances [33, 36].

Diffuse lamellar keratitis (Sands of Sahara syndrome) is a sterile inflammation probably caused by the introduction of toxins in the flap interface [37, 38]. It is graded in four stages, with stage one and two being mild and visually unthreatening, while stage four can lead to corneal melting and permanent changes [33, 39]. In comparison to diffuse lamellar keratitis, central toxic keratopathy is a rare noninflammatory central corneal opacification linked to enzymatic degradation of keratocytes with spontaneous resolution and mild central opacification which often causes refractory hyperopic shift [40].

Pressure-induced stromal keratitis is also easily mistaken with diffuse lamellar keratitis but is caused by postoperative steroid use which leads to increase in intraocular pressure and represents as cystoid lamellar edema [41].

Infectious keratitis after LASIK is extremely rare but can be quite serious since invading organisms are already implanted into the deep corneal stroma. The most often isolated organisms include *Streptococcus pneumoniae*, *Staphylococcus aureus*, *Mycobacterium chelonae*, and *Nocardia asteroides* [33, 42].

Epithelial ingrowth under the LASIK flap is reported to occur in merely 1–2% of patients and is caused by migration of epithelial cells under the flap. It is usually insignificant, but if epithelial cells continue to grow, it can cause flap distortion and melting causing visual disturbances [43].

Late postoperative complications include dry eye, night vision problems, corneal haze, regression of refractive error, and iatrogenic corneal ectasia.

Dry eye syndrome is caused by denervation and cutting of nerve fibers during the formation of the flap, removal of corneal tissue by excimer laser, and changes in the shape of the cornea. Dry eye syndrome is usually transient and symptoms fade away after healing period. It causes discomfort, fluctuation in vision quality, slower healing, and epithelial damage and may lead to regression of refractive error and reduced vision quality [44].

Symptoms of impaired visual quality are usually more expressed during the night due to physiological pupil dilatation. The main causes of nighttime issues are the increase in spherical aberrations at the centrally flatted cornea, decentered ablations, too small optical zones, newly emerging lens opacities, and induced astigmatism [45].

Corneal haze reduces corneal transparency at variable degrees and is more common after PRK and correction of high myopia (>−6.00 D). Besides the ablation depth, it is correlated with an excessive ocular UV-B radiation, duration of the epithelial defect, postoperative steroid treatment, male sex, and certain population with brown iris [46].

Regression of refractive error is defined as return of part of the primary refractive error and is associated with increase in thickness and curvature of the cornea. Potential mechanisms include nuclear sclerosis, stromal synthesis (wound healing), compensatory epithelial hyperplasia, and iatrogenic keratectasia [47].

Postoperative ectasia is linked to biomechanical weakening of the cornea and is characterized with progressive corneal steepening, either centrally or inferiorly, resulting in severe progressive irregular astigmatism and decrease of both uncorrected and best-corrected visual acuity. The incidence of ectasia after LASIK has been estimated between 0.04 and 0.9% [48]. Risk factors include abnormal topographic findings, thin cornea, and high myopia together with young age at the time of surgery [49].

Intraoperative complications of SMILE procedure are usually not sight threatening, and the procedure usually can be continued [13, 15, 50]. The most common complications are incision or cap tears, suction loss, cap perforation, black spots, and opaque bubble layer which lead to cap lenticular adhesions and retained lenticule. Regarding the postoperative complications of SMILE procedure, they are similar to all laser refractive procedures and include epithelial ingrowth, dry eye, diffuse lamellar keratitis, corneal haze, irregular astigmatism, minor interface infiltrates, increased aberrations, and iatrogenic ectasia [50, 51].

3. Intraocular correction of myopia

Two basic intraocular procedures exist: phakic intraocular lens (pIOL) implantation and refractive lens exchange (RLE) with posterior chamber IOL implantation.

3.1 Phakic intraocular lenses

Phakic intraocular lenses (pIOL) provide a safe and effective alternative for young patients with moderate to high refractive errors who may not be suitable candidates for excimer laser procedures or who prefer a reversible form of vision correction with efficacy comparable to results of LASIK [52]. It has been established that attempted corrections of high myopia with excimer laser procedures induce more higher-order aberrations, affecting vision quality and creating problems such as glare, halos, and ghost imaging [53]. Additional advantages of intraocular procedures are a broader range of treatable ametropia, faster visual recovery, more stable refraction, and better visual quality. In addition, the pIOL implantation does not affect accommodation, and the procedure is reversible [52, 54].

Currently, there are two types of phakic intraocular lenses approved for correcting refractive errors: anterior chamber—iris fixated—and posterior chamber. Verisyse and Veriflex lenses are iris-fixated intraocular lenses. More than 160,000 of these lenses have been safely implanted worldwide [55]. The Verisyse pIOL is made from rigid, ultraviolet-absorbing polymethyl methacrylate (PMMA). This lens requires a 5.5–6.5-mm incision, depending on the optic size of the lens, whereas the Veriflex pIOL requires a 3.2-mm incision. The Verisyse pIOL is available for myopia, hypermetropia, and astigmatism. For myopia, the pIOL is available in powers from −1.00 to −23.50 D in 0.50 D steps with two optic diameters of 5.0 or 6.0 mm. The Veriflex pIOL is a foldable implant with 6.0 mm flexible optic made of hydrophobic polysiloxane and features a PMMA haptic. It is available only for myopia in powers ranging from −2.00 to −14.50 D in 0.50 D steps.

The Visian Implantable Collamer Lens (ICL) is a posterior chamber phakic intraocular lens resting in the ciliary sulcus. ICL is made from soft advanced collamer material and requires 3.2 mm incision. It is available for myopia, hypermetropia, and astigmatism. For myopia, the pIOL is available in powers from −0.50 to −18.00 D in 0.50 D steps with four lens diameters (12.1, 12.6, 13.2, 13.6 mm) and optical zone up to 6.1 mm.

3.1.1 Preoperative examination and indications for phakic intraocular lens implantation

The preoperative evaluation of a patient for pIOL is the same as for any kind of refractive procedure. Inclusion criteria are more than 21 years of age, refractive stability (<0.50 D of change) for at least 1 year, ACD ≥ 3.0 mm measured from endothelium, endothelial cell count >2300 cells/mm^2 (>2500 cell/mm^2 if <40 years of age, > 2000 cells/mm^2 if >40 years of age), irido-corneal angle ≥30° (at least grade II by gonioscopy examination), mesopic pupil size <6.00 mm, no anomaly of iris or pupil function, no evolving retinal pathology, absence of uveitis or any kind of ocular inflammation, and absence of glaucoma or any systemic immunological disorder [56, 57].

3.1.2 Intraocular lens power calculation and diameter selection

pIOL optic power is calculated with the software provided by the manufacturer. The calculation is based on the formula developed by van der Heijde [58]. The formula uses the patient's refraction at the 12-mm spectacle plane or the vertex refraction, the corneal keratometry dioptric power at its apex, and central ACD [59]. For Verisyse and Veriflex lenses, only one lens diameter is available, while for the ICL overall diameter depends on the ciliary sulcus diameter and should provide perfect stability with no excess of compression forces to the sulcus and allow correct vaulting. The ICL's diameter should be oversized 0.5–1.0 mm from the white-to-white (WTW) measurements in myopic eyes and the same length or oversized 0.5 mm in hyperopic eyes. The internal diameter of the ciliary sulcus can be measured by ultrasound biometry (UBM) or can be approximated by horizontal WTW measurement obtained manually using a caliper or automatically by topographic or biometric devices [60].

3.1.3 Limitations and possible complications of phakic intraocular lenses

The complications relating to pIOLs can, at times, be more disabling than those from keratorefractive surgery. Night vision problems, corneal decompensation, glaucoma, cataract formation, dyscoria, uveitis, and endophthalmitis are potential complications after pIOL implantation. Night vision problems such as glare, halos, and diplopia are related to decentration of the pIOL and/or an optic diameter that is too small relative to the pupil size [61].

Surgically induced astigmatism is an issue primarily correlated with rigid Verisyse lenses and incision diameter. However, some investigators reported that the resulting surgically induced astigmatism (SIA) was less than expected [62, 63]. However, when compared with the Veriflex pIOL and ICL, the SIA was significantly higher [64].

Implantation of a pIOL, whether iris fixated or positioned in the posterior chamber, is associated with an accelerated decrease in endothelial cell density (ECD) [60]. Damage to the corneal endothelium may be due to the direct contact between pIOL and the inner surface of the cornea during implantation, from postoperative changes in pIOL position, or from subclinical inflammation, and direct toxicity to the endothelium. The magnitude of ECD loss after phakic intraocular lens implantation surpasses the expected natural annual decrease of 0.6% as reported in a 1997 benchmark study based on 42 adults [65]. Following implantation of an iris-claw phakic intraocular lens, the loss of ECD is highest during the first year varying between 0.75 and 7.2% [66]. Thereafter, the ECD loss continues without following an obvious pattern, to about 8.9% after 10 years. However, with an ICL the impact on the endothelium is claimed to be lower because the implant is placed in the posterior chamber further away from the endothelium itself. For the ICL the ECD loss is about 1.7% after 2 years [60] increasing to 6.2% after 8 years [54] and up to 19.75% after 12 years [67].

In our experience after ICL implantation, there is a linear decrease in ECD over a 3-year period, without any signs of exponential EC loss or reaching a plateau or stable ECD during this time (**Figure 5**).

With modern pIOL designs, increased intraocular pressure (IOP) seems to be relatively uncommon after 3 months postoperatively and is typically thought to be related to corticosteroid response [68]. Posterior chamber pIOLs cause narrowing of anterior chamber angle due to its position in ciliary sulcus, and its sizing (too long lenses which cause excessive vaulting >750 μm) is closely correlated with possible angle-closure glaucoma, pupillary block glaucoma, or pigmentary dispersion glaucoma [69, 70]. Given the risk of pupillary block, peripheral iridectomy or iridotomy is carried out as a preventative measure in anterior pIOL procedures, while in newer models of ICL with aquaport, technology is not needed.

Pupil ovalization/iris retraction is mainly correlated with iris-fixated pIOL and can occur if fixation of the pIOL haptics is performed asymmetrically [61, 68, 71]. No progressive pupil ovalization has been reported.

Formation of cataract due to the iris-claw pIOL is unlikely because the pIOL is inserted over a miotic pupil without contact with the crystalline lens [61]. The incidence of cataract formation was 1.1% for the iris-fixated pIOL. The overall incidence of cataract formation for posterior chamber pIOLs was 9.60%, which is significantly higher in comparison to iris-fixated pIOLs [72]. With various generations of the ICL, appearance of cataract formation is different. The less vaulted

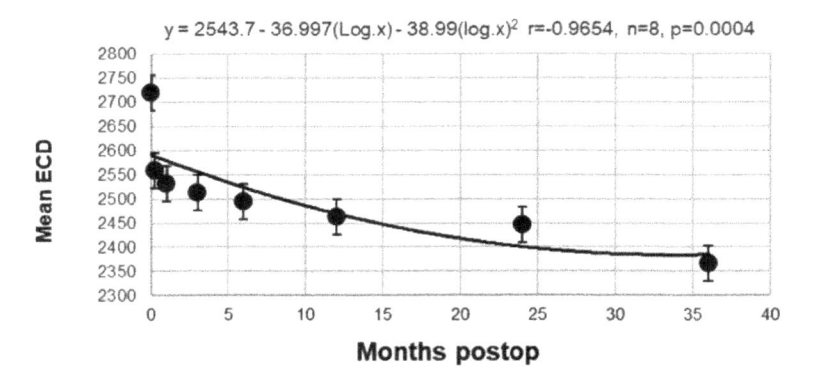

Figure 5.
Mean endothelial cell density during the 3-year follow-up (28 eyes); ± SD error bars are included indicating the variance in the data.

model V3 caused a higher incidence of cataract formation than the newer V4 and V5 models [73]. With the V4 model, the recently published FDA study showed an incidence of 2.1% anterior subcapsular opacities, which is the most common type of cataract after pIOL [59]. Possible reasons are operative trauma, continuous or intermittent contact of the posterior chamber pIOL with the crystalline lens, insufficient nutrition through anterior chamber flow between the posterior chamber pIOL and the crystalline lens, and chronic subclinical inflammation with disruption of the blood-aqueous barrier due to friction between the pIOL and posterior iris or the haptic on the ciliary sulcus [74–76].

The risk of uveitis is a concern given the proximity of pIOLs to the iris, but it does not seem to be a significant long-term complication with modern designs. With iris-fixated pIOLs, a difficulty with enclavation of the iris can lead to iris atrophy and decentration of the implant [52]. Retinal detachment seems to be uncommon and lower than in clear lens extraction cases [68, 77]. A few cases of endophthalmitis have been reported after pIOL implantation, but it seems less common after pIOL implantation and then after cataract surgery [78, 79].

3.2 Refractive lens exchange

Refractive lens exchange (RLE) is by definition used to indicate the replacement of the cataractous/clear crystalline lens with an intraocular lens (IOL) to achieve emmetropia/near emmetropia. The improved efficacy, predictability, and safety of modern-day phacoemulsification have resulted in a resurgence of lens extraction as a modality for correction of high myopia. Increased numbers of RLE are being performed worldwide, especially in patients not suitable for LASIK or pIOL or with early lens changes in the presbyopia age group [80, 81]. Optics of the IOL confer better quality of vision as compared with LASIK, and this optical quality does not degrade with time except in the presence of a posterior capsular opacification. The refractive results are predictable and stable with a larger range of refractive correction possible than with either LASIK or pIOL. RLE addresses refractive error and cataract and with the use of modern multifocal IOLs results in a significant degree of spectacle independence for the patient. Visual recovery is faster, and it is more cost-effective, as the higher cost of pIOLs and future cataract surgery is eliminated. The principles of surgery are in the domain of most cataract/anterior segment surgeons [82].

Overall, patient satisfaction scores after implantation of multifocal IOLs are high. For example, using a 0–10 self-recording analogue scale, you can expect

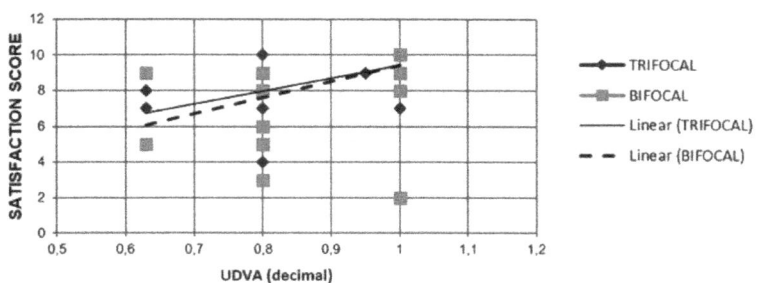

Figure 6.
Postoperative uncorrected distance visual acuity and patient satisfaction after RLE with implantation of multifocal IOLs.

typical average satisfaction scores of 8.8 (Zeiss bifocal IOL, n = 48, range 2–10) and 9.00 (Zeiss trifocal IOL, n = 52, range 4–10). On closer examination satisfaction scores are closely linked to post-op uncorrected distance and intermediate, visual acuity as demonstrated in **Figure 6**.

Advanced technology multifocal IOLs tend to be less forgiving with respect to the surgical technique, multifocal IOL power selection, ocular comorbidities, and patient selection. Comorbidities such as dry eye, vitreomacular pathology, or implant decentration may be tolerated in patients after a monofocal IOL implantation. However, these are much less tolerated by the multifocal IOL patients [83, 84].

Presbyopia-correcting intraocular lenses should provide post-op emmetropia for the best visual outcome, as small amounts of residual refractive errors can limit visual performance and jeopardize the result [85].

3.2.1 Preoperative examination and indications for refractive lens exchange

In evaluating the highly myopic patient, several aspects apart from the routine cataract/refractive surgery assessment should be noted. A detailed past ocular history is important, as previous refractive surgery or phakic intraocular lens implants or retinal problems (e.g., vitrectomy for previous retinal detachment) will affect lens formula choices and their final prognosis. Preoperative assessment should also include a detailed clinical examination of their lens status (e.g., cataract density and any zonular weakness) and refraction status of both eyes, as well as a dilated examination of the fovea and periphery for any retina disorder (e.g., myopic choroidal neovascular membrane, macular schisis, retinal tears, or detachment). Other issues for discussion include the potential use of toric or multifocal IOLs. Ideally, a larger haptic platform toric lens should be used in high myopes to reduce the risk of postoperative lens rotation, as the capsular bag is often large and floppy. In some cases, the use of a capsular tension ring to stretch the capsular bag may be required to prevent rotations. Multifocal IOLs should only be used in an eye with no retinal disorder [86].

Inclusion criteria are more than 40 years of age with myopia not amenable to conventional laser refractive surgery (e.g., high refractive error, corneal irregularities, thin cornea) or phakic IOLS (e.g., shallow anterior chamber, poor endothelial cell count, early cataract changes), presbyopic myopic patients who want reasonable independence from glasses for both distance, and near-vision, myopic patients with early lens changes who desire refractive correction [80, 86]. For multifocal IOL it is important to rule out any irregularities of iris or pupil function, evolving retinal pathology, absence of uveitis, or any kind of ocular inflammation.

3.2.2 Limitations and possible complications of refractive lens exchange

The commonest disadvantage is the loss of accommodation with the need for near-vision glasses in the cases of monofocal IOL and the inherent risk associated with intraocular surgery, especially in high myopes [80]. The risk for endophthalmitis in general cataract surgery with implantation of a posterior chamber IOL is 0.1–0.7% with an optimal antiseptic perioperative treatment regimen [87]. Lens surgery is significantly more challenging in a highly myopic eye for several reasons. The issues that we take for granted in an eye of normal length (22–25 mm) such as the accuracy of axial length measurements and the choice of lens formula become a significant issue in the highly myopic eye as the predicted refractive outcomes are not achieved consistently. Axial length measurement error has been largely overcome by the use of optical interferometry. Despite this, consistent hyperopic errors are still reported. Improved predictive results are obtained with the Barrett Universal II (software constants), Haigis (ULIB), SRK/T, Holladay 2 (software constants), and Olsen (software constants) formulas in eyes with axial lengths greater than 26.0 mm and IOL powers greater than 6.0 D. In the eyes with axial lengths greater than 26.0 mm and IOL less than 6.00 D, the Barrett Universal II formula (software constants) and the Haigis (axial length adjusted) and Holladay 1 formulas (axial length adjusted) should be used [88, 89].

Intraoperatively, a highly myopic eye is surgically more challenging as the anterior chamber is deeper, with a floppy and large capsular bag and occasionally zonular weakness [90]. The anterior chamber is often unstable, and it is even less stable in a previously vitrectomized high myopic patient. There is also a concern that with elongated axial lengths, there is a higher risk of bag instability that can cause impaired vision, and the more complicated the IOL design is, the more sensitive the IOL is to final centration. A study by Soda et al. found that in uncomplicated cataract surgery with an IOL in the bag, the maximum decentration can be 0.3 mm for a satisfying result [91]. In addition, it is reported that myopic patients may exhibit worse results with more reported subjective symptoms and measurable aberrations like coma and glare in mesopic and scotopic lighting conditions compared to non-myopic controls, after multifocal IOL implantation with approximately the same amount of decentration [91]. RLE may increase the risk for retinal detachment and is generally not considered in myopic pre-presbyopic patients who can still accommodate.

The incidence of retinal detachment is especially high among younger age groups (<50 years) and in the eyes with long axial length > 26 mm. The reported incidence of retinal detachment after RLE ranges from 2 to 8%. Meticulous surgery with minimal intraoperative vitreous disturbance and a regular follow-up postoperatively until the occurrence of posterior vitreous detachment can reduce the risk of retinal detachment further. With the higher risk of retinal detachment in younger patients, it is prudent to defer RLE in patients younger than 40 years if possible [92].

Other possible causes of unfavorable visual outcome after uncomplicated phacoemulsification are cystoid macular edema (CME) and choroidal neovascular membrane (CNVM). Overall incidence of subclinical CME diagnosed with optical coherence tomography (OCT) is 5%, and incidence of clinical CME is 3%; however, high myopia does not increase the risk of CME [93]. Reported incidence of CNVM after RLE for myopia is 12.5% [94]; however, whether this was related to the higher degree of myopia with preexisting lacquer crack that was missed or due to some inflammatory mediators and free radicals released after surgery cannot be conclusively proved. Because the reported incidence of CNVM after uncomplicated phacoemulsification is not high, we assume that it is secondary to the degree of myopia, and it is prudent to perform OCT preoperatively in all RLE patients, especially those with more than 10 D of myopia. The presence of a myopic CNVM in the fellow eye is also considered as a risk factor for developing CNVM in the operated eye [80, 94].

4. Conclusions

Surgical treatment of myopia is a viable, safe, efficient, and predictable method for treating patients with myopia. There are several options of surgical treatment; we as doctors must always use our best judgment and available data to make sure we recommend the best method for each patient and their respective needs while taking into account any possible risk and contraindications. Among elective procedures in medicine, myopia treatment is one of the most commonly performed surgeries because of the positive effect it brings the patients' quality of life.

Author details

Maja Bohac[1,2*], Maja Pauk Gulic[1,2], Alma Biscevic[1,2] and Ivan Gabric[1,2]

1 Specialty Eye Hospital Svjetlost, Zagreb, Croatia

2 School of Medicine, University of Rijeka, Croatia

*Address all correspondence to: maja.bohac@svjetlost.hr

IntechOpen

© 2019 The Author(s). Licensee IntechOpen. This chapter is distributed under the terms of the Creative Commons Attribution License (http://creativecommons.org/licenses/by/3.0), which permits unrestricted use, distribution, and reproduction in any medium, provided the original work is properly cited.

References

[1] Fan DSP, Rao SK, Cheung EYY, Islam M, Chew S, Lam DSC. Astigmatism in Chinese preschool children: Prevalence, change, and effect on refractive development. The British Journal of Ophthalmology. 2004;**88**: 938-941. DOI: 10.1136/bjo.2003.030338

[2] Dolgin E. The myopia boom. Nature. 2015;**519**:276-278. DOI: 10.1038/519276a

[3] Holden BA, Fricke TR, Wilson DA, Jong M, Naidoo KS, Sankaridurg P, et al. Global prevalence of myopia and high myopia and temporal trends from 2000 through 2050. Ophthalmology. 2016;**123**:1036-1042. DOI: 10.1016/j.ophtha.2016.01.006

[4] Reinstein DZ, Archer TJ, Gobbe M. The history of LASIK. Journal of Refractive Surgery. 2012;**28**:291-298. DOI: 10.3928/1081597X-20120229-01

[5] Ehlers N, Hjortdal JO. Excimer laser refractive keratectomy for high myopia. 6-month follow-up of patients treated bilaterally. Acta Ophthalmologica. 1992;**70**:578-586

[6] Rosman M, Alió JL, Ortiz D, Perez-Santonja JJ. Comparison of LASIK and photorefractive keratectomy for myopia from −10.00 to −18.00 diopters 10 years after surgery. Journal of Refractive Surgery. 2010;**26**:168-176. DOI: 10.3928/1081597X-20100224-02

[7] Sia RK, Coe CD, Edwards JD, Ryan DS, Bower KS. Visual outcomes after Epi-LASIK and PRK for low and moderate myopia. Journal of Refractive Surgery. 2012;**28**:65-71. DOI: 10.3928/1081597X-20111004-01

[8] Ambrósio R, Wilson S. LASIK vs LASEK vs PRK: Advantages and indications. Seminars in Ophthalmology. 2003;**18**:2-10

[9] Ghadhfan F, Al-Rajhi A, Wagoner MD. Laser in situ keratomileusis versus surface ablation: Visual outcomes and complications. Journal of Cataract and Refractive Surgery. 2007;**33**:2041-2048. DOI: 10.1016/j.jcrs.2007.07.026

[10] Hofmeister EM, Bishop FM, Kaupp SE, Schallhorn SC. Randomized dose-response analysis of mitomycin-C to prevent haze after photorefractive keratectomy for high myopia. Journal of Cataract and Refractive Surgery. 2013;**39**:1358-1365. DOI: 10.1016/j.jcrs.2013.03.029

[11] Gimbel HV, DeBroff BM, Beldavs RA, van Westenbrugge JA, Ferensowicz M. Comparison of laser and manual removal of corneal epithelium for photorefractive keratectomy. Journal of Refractive Surgery. 1995;**11**:36-41

[12] von Jagow B, Kohnen T. Corneal architecture of femtosecond laser and microkeratome flaps imaged by anterior segment optical coherence tomography. Journal of Cataract and Refractive Surgery. 2009;**35**:35-41. DOI: 10.1016/j.jcrs.2008.09.013

[13] Reinstein DZ, Archer TJ, Randleman JB. Mathematical model to compare the relative tensile strength of the cornea after PRK, LASIK, and small incision lenticule extraction. Journal of Refractive Surgery. 2013;**29**:454-460. DOI: 10.3928/1081597X-20130617-03

[14] Guerin MB, Darcy F, O'Connor J, O'Keeffe M. Excimer laser photorefractive keratectomy for low to moderate myopia using a 5.0 mm treatment zone and no transitional zone: 16-year follow-up. Journal of Cataract and Refractive Surgery. 2012;**38**(7):1246-1250. DOI: 10.1016/j.jcrs.2012.03.027

[15] Sekundo W, Kunert KS, Blum M. Small incision corneal refractive surgery using the small incision lenticule extraction (SMILE) procedure for the correction of myopia and myopic

astigmatism: Results of a 6 month prospective study. The British Journal of Ophthalmology. 2011;**95**:335-339. DOI: 10.1136/bjo.2009.174284

[16] Wu D, Wang Y, Zhang L, Wei S, Tang X. Corneal biomechanical effects: Small-incision lenticule extraction versus femtosecond laser-assisted laser in situ keratomileusis. Journal of Cataract and Refractive Surgery. 2014;**40**:954-962. DOI: 10.1016/j.jcrs.2013.07.056

[17] Thompson V, Gordon M. Use of the excimer laser in refractive surgery. Seminars in Ophthalmology. 1994;**9**:91-96

[18] Carr J, Hersh P, Tsubota K. Patient evaluation for refractive surgery. In: Azar D, editor. Refractive Surgery. 2nd ed. Philadelphia: Elsevier Inc.; 2007. pp. 81-88. DOI: 10.1016/B978-0-323-03599-6.50068-7

[19] Morse JS, Schallhorn SC, Hettinger K, Tanzer D. Role of depressive symptoms in patient satisfaction with visual quality after laser in situ keratomileusis. Journal of Cataract and Refractive Surgery. 2009;**35**:341-346. DOI: 10.1016/j.jcrs.2008.10.046

[20] Nourouzi H, Rajavi J, Okhovatpour MA. Time to resolution of corneal edema after long-term contact lens wear. American Journal of Ophthalmology. 2006;**142**:671-673. DOI: 10.1016/j.ajo.2006.04.061

[21] Chuck RS, Jacobs DS, Lee JK, Afshari NA, Vitale S, Shen TT, et al. Refractive errors and refractive surgery preferred practice pattern®. Ophthalmology. 2018;**125**:P1-P104. DOI: 10.1016/j.ophtha.2017.10.003

[22] Cua IY, Pepose JS. Late corneal scarring after photorefractive keratectomy concurrent with development of systemic lupus erythematosus. Journal of Refractive Surgery. 2002;**18**:750-752

[23] Simpson RG, Moshirfar M, Edmonds JN, Christiansen SM, Behunin N. Laser in situ keratomileusis in patients with collagen vascular disease: A review of the literature. Clinical Ophthalmology. 2012;**6**:1827-1837. DOI: 10.2147/OPTH.S36690

[24] Fraunfelder FW, Rich LF. Laser-assisted in situ keratomileusis complications in diabetes mellitus. Cornea. 2002;**21**:246-248

[25] Sharma S, Rekha W, Sharma T, Downey G. Refractive issues in pregnancy. The Australian & New Zealand Journal of Obstetrics & Gynaecology. 2006;**46**:186-188. DOI: 10.1111/j.1479-828X.2006.00569.x

[26] Seiler T, Koufala K, Richter G. Iatrogenic keratectasia after laser in situ keratomileusis. Journal of Refractive Surgery. 1998;**14**:312-317

[27] Hodge C, Lawless M, Sutton G. Keratectasia following LASIK in a patient with uncomplicated PRK in the fellow eye. Journal of Cataract and Refractive Surgery. 2011;**37**:603-607. DOI: 10.1016/j.jcrs.2010.12.036

[28] Randleman JB, Woodward M, Lynn MJ, Stulting RD. Risk assessment for ectasia after corneal refractive surgery. Ophthalmology. 2008;**115**:37-50. DOI: 10.1016/j.ophtha.2007.03.073

[29] Santhiago MR, Smadja D, Wilson SE, Krueger RR, Monteiro MLR, Randleman JB. Role of percent tissue altered on ectasia after LASIK in eyes with suspicious topography. Journal of Refractive Surgery. 2015;**31**:258-265. DOI: 10.3928/1081597X-20150319-05

[30] Cobo-Soriano R, Beltrán J, Baviera J. LASIK outcomes in patients with underlying systemic contraindications: A preliminary study. Ophthalmology. 2006;**113**. DOI: 1118. e1-8. doi:10.1016/j.ophtha.2006.02.023

[31] Arora T, Sharma N, Arora S, Titiyal JS. Fulminant herpetic keratouveitis with flap necrosis following laser in situ keratomileusis: Case report and review of literature. Journal of Cataract and Refractive Surgery. 2014;**40**:2152-2156. DOI: 10.1016/j.jcrs.2014.09.018

[32] Ahn H, Kim J-K, Kim CK, Han GH, Seo KY, Kim EK, et al. Comparison of laser in situ keratomileusis flaps created by 3 femtosecond lasers and a microkeratome. Journal of Cataract and Refractive Surgery. 2011;**37**:349-357. DOI: 10.1016/j.jcrs.2010.08.042

[33] Farah S, Ghanem R, Azar D. LASIK complications and their management. In: Azar D, editor. Refractive Surgery. 2nd ed. Philadelphia: Elsevier Inc.; 2007. pp. 195-221

[34] Rush SW, Cofoid P, Rush RB. Incidence and outcomes of anterior chamber gas bubble during femtosecond flap creation for laser-assisted in situ keratomileusis. Journal of Ophthalmology. 2015;**2015**:542127. DOI: 10.1155/2015/542127

[35] Stonecipher KG, Dishler JG, Ignacio TS, Binder PS. Transient light sensitivity after femtosecond laser flap creation: Clinical findings and management. Journal of Cataract and Refractive Surgery. 2006;**32**:91-94. DOI: 10.1016/j.jcrs.2005.11.015

[36] Carpel EF, Carlson KH, Shannon S. Folds and striae in laser in situ keratomileusis flaps. Journal of Refractive Surgery. 1999;**15**:687-690

[37] Samuel MA, Kaufman SC, Ahee JA, Wee C, Bogorad D. Diffuse lamellar keratitis associated with carboxymethylcellulose sodium 1% after laser in situ keratomileusis. Journal of Cataract and Refractive Surgery. 2002;**28**:1409-1411

[38] Kaufman SC. Post-LASIK interface keratitis, Sands of the Sahara syndrome, and microkeratome blades. Journal of Cataract and Refractive Surgery. 1999;**25**:603-604

[39] Linebarger EJ, Hardten DR, Lindstrom RL. Diffuse lamellar keratitis: Diagnosis and management. Journal of Cataract and Refractive Surgery. 2000;**26**:1072-1077

[40] Sonmez B, Maloney RK. Central toxic keratopathy: Description of a syndrome in laser refractive surgery. American Journal of Ophthalmology. 2007;**143**:420-427.e2. DOI: 10.1016/J.AJO.2006.11.019

[41] Miyai T, Yonemura T, Nejima R, Otani S, Miyata K, Amano S. Interlamellar flap edema due to steroid-induced ocular hypertension after laser in situ keratomileusis. Japanese Journal of Ophthalmology. 2007. DOI: 10.1007/s10384-006-0441-y

[42] Llovet F, de Rojas V, Interlandi E, Martín C, Cobo-Soriano R, Ortega-Usobiaga J, et al. Infectious keratitis in 204 586 LASIK procedures. Ophthalmology. 2010;**117**:232.e1-4-238.e1-4. DOI: 10.1016/j.ophtha.2009.07.011

[43] Caster AI, Friess DW, Schwendeman FJ. Incidence of epithelial ingrowth in primary and retreatment laser in situ keratomileusis. Journal of Cataract and Refractive Surgery. 2010;**36**:97-101. DOI: 10.1016/j.jcrs.2009.07.039

[44] Albietz JM, Lenton LM, McLennan SG, McLennan SG. Chronic dry eye and regression after laser in situ keratomileusis for myopia. Journal of Cataract and Refractive Surgery. 2004;**30**:675-684. DOI: 10.1016/j.jcrs.2003.07.003

[45] Myung D, Schallhorn S, Manche EE. Pupil size and LASIK: A review. Journal of Refractive Surgery. 2013;**29**:734-741. DOI: 10.3928/1081597X-20131021-02

[46] Alió JL, Muftuoglu O, Ortiz D, Artola A, Pérez-Santonja JJ, de Luna GC, et al. Ten-year follow-up of photorefractive keratectomy for myopia of more than −6 diopters. American Journal of Ophthalmology. 2008;**145**: 37-45. DOI: 10.1016/j.ajo.2007.09.009

[47] Alió JL, Soria F, Abbouda A, Peña-García P. Laser in situ keratomileusis for −6.00 to −18.00 diopters of myopia and up to −5.00 diopters of astigmatism: 15-year follow-up. Journal of Cataract and Refractive Surgery. 2015;**41**:33-40. DOI: 10.1016/j.jcrs.2014.08.029

[48] Santhiago MR, Giacomin NT, Smadja D, Bechara SJ. Ectasia risk factors in refractive surgery. Clinical Ophthalmology. 2016;**10**:713-720. DOI: 10.2147/OPTH.S51313

[49] Giri P, Azar DT. Risk profiles of ectasia after keratorefractive surgery. Current Opinion in Ophthalmology. 2017;**28**:337-342. DOI: 10.1097/ICU.0000000000000383

[50] Chan C, Lawless M, Sutton G, Versace P, Hodge C. Small incision lenticule extraction (SMILE) in 2015. Clinical and Experimental Optometry. 2016;**99**:204-212. DOI: 10.1111/cxo.12380

[51] Ivarsen A, Hjortdal JØ. Topography-guided photorefractive keratectomy for irregular astigmatism after small incision lenticule extraction. Journal of Refractive Surgery. 2014;**30**:429-432. DOI: 10.3928/1081597X-20140508-02

[52] Huang D, Schallhorn SC, Sugar A, Farjo AA, Majmudar PA, Trattler WB, et al. Phakic intraocular lens implantation for the correction of myopiaa report by the American Academy of Ophthalmology. Ophthalmology. 2009;**116**:2244-2258. DOI: 10.1016/j.ophtha.2009.08.018

[53] Applegate RA, Howland HC. Refractive surgery, optical aberrations, and visual performance. Journal of Refractive Surgery. 1997;**13**:295-299

[54] Igarashi A, Shimizu K, Kamiya K. Eight-year follow-up of posterior chamber phakic intraocular lens implantation for moderate to high myopia. American Journal of Ophthalmology. 2014;**157**:532-539.e1. DOI: 10.1016/j.ajo.2013.11.006

[55] Ghanem R, Azer D. Phakic intraocular lenses. In: Yanoff M, Augsburger JJ, editors. Ophthalmology. Edinburgh: Mosby, Elsevier; 2009, p. 186

[56] Pineda-Fernández A, Jaramillo J, Vargas J, Jaramillo M, Jaramillo J, Galíndez A. Phakic posterior chamber intraocular lens for high myopia. Journal of Cataract and Refractive Surgery. 2004;**30**:2277-2283. DOI: 10.1016/j.jcrs.2004.03.035

[57] Javitt JC, Tielsch JM, Canner JK, Kolb MM, Sommer A, Steinberg EP. National outcomes of cataract extraction. Increased risk of retinal complications associated with Nd:YAG laser capsulotomy. The Cataract Patient Outcomes Research Team. Ophthalmology. 1992;**99**:1487-1497; discussion 1497-8

[58] Van Der Heijde GL. Some optical aspects of implantation of an IOL in a myopic eye. European Journal of Implant Refractive Surgery. 1989;**1**:245-248. DOI: 10.1016/S0955-3681(89)80082-6

[59] Sanders DR, Vukich JA, Doney K, Gaston M, Implantable Contact Lens in Treatment of Myopia Study Group. U.S. Food and Drug Administration clinical trial of the Implantable Contact Lens for moderate to high myopia. Ophthalmology. 2003;**110**:255-266

[60] Goukon H, Kamiya K, Shimizu K, Igarashi A. Comparison of corneal endothelial cell density and morphology after posterior chamber phakic

intraocular lens implantation with and without a central hole. The British Journal of Ophthalmology. 2017;**101**:1461-1465. DOI: 10.1136/bjophthalmol-2016-309363

[61] Kohnen T, Kook D, Morral M, Güell JL. Phakic intraocular lenses: Part 2: Results and complications. Journal of Cataract and Refractive Surgery. 2010;**36**:2168-2194. DOI: 10.1016/j.jcrs.2010.10.007

[62] Alió JL, Mulet ME, Shalaby AMM. Artisan phakic iris claw intraocular lens for high primary and secondary hyperopia. Journal of Refractive Surgery. 2002;**18**:697-707

[63] Menezo JL, Aviño JA, Cisneros A, Rodriguez-Salvador V, Martinez-Costa R. Iris claw phakic intraocular lens for high myopia. Journal of Refractive Surgery. 1997;**13**:545-555

[64] Coullet J, Guëll J-L, Fournié P, Grandjean H, Gaytan J, Arné J-L, et al. Iris-supported phakic lenses (rigid vs foldable version) for treating moderately high myopia: Randomized paired eye comparison. American Journal of Ophthalmology. 2006;**142**:909-916. DOI: 10.1016/j.ajo.2006.07.021

[65] Bourne WM, Nelson LR, Hodge DO. Central corneal endothelial cell changes over a ten-year period. Investigative Ophthalmology and Visual Science. 1997;**38**:779-782

[66] Chebli S, Rabilloud M, Burillon C, Kocaba V. Corneal endothelial tolerance after iris-fixated phakic intraocular lens implantation: A model to predict endothelial cell survival. Cornea. 2018;**37**:591-595. DOI: 10.1097/ICO.0000000000001527

[67] Moya T, Javaloy J, Montés-Micó R, Beltrán J, Muñoz G, Montalbán R. Implantable collamer lens for myopia: Assessment 12 years after implantation. Journal of Refractive Surgery. 2015;**31**:548-556. DOI: 10.3928/1081597X-20150727-05

[68] Stulting RD, John ME, Maloney RK, Assil KK, Arrowsmith PN, Thompson VM, et al. Three-year results of Artisan/Verisyse phakic intraocular lens implantation. Results of the United States Food And Drug Administration clinical trial. Ophthalmology. 2008;**115**:464-472, e1. DOI: 10.1016/j.ophtha.2007.08.039

[69] Hoyos JE, Dementiev DD, Cigales M, Hoyos-Chacón J, Hoffer KJ. Phakic refractive lens experience in Spain. Journal of Cataract and Refractive Surgery. 2002;**28**:1939-1946

[70] García-Feijoó J, Alfaro IJ, Cuiña-Sardiña R, Méndez-Hernandez C, Del Castillo JMB, García-Sánchez J. Ultrasound biomicroscopy examination of posterior chamber phakic intraocular lens position. Ophthalmology. 2003;**110**:163-172

[71] Maloney RK, Nguyen LH, John ME. Artisan phakic intraocular lens for myopia: Short-term results of a prospective, multicenter study. Ophthalmology. 2002;**109**:1631-1641

[72] Chen L-J, Chang Y-J, Kuo JC, Rajagopal R, Azar DT. Metaanalysis of cataract development after phakic intraocular lens surgery. Journal of Cataract and Refractive Surgery. 2008;**34**:1181-1200. DOI: 10.1016/j.jcrs.2008.03.029

[73] Menezo JL, Peris-Martínez C, Cisneros A, Martínez-Costa R. Posterior chamber phakic intraocular lenses to correct high myopia: A comparative study between Staar and Adatomed models. Journal of Refractive Surgery. 2001;**17**:32-42

[74] Gonvers M, Bornet C, Othenin-Girard P. Implantable contact lens for moderate to high myopia: Relationship

of vaulting to cataract formation. Journal of Cataract Refractive Surgery. 2003;**29**:918-924

[75] Sánchez-Galeana CA, Smith RJ, Sanders DR, Rodríguez FX, Litwak S, Montes M, et al. Lens opacities after posterior chamber phakic intraocular lens implantation. Ophthalmology. 2003;**110**:781-785

[76] Lackner B, Pieh S, Schmidinger G, Hanselmayer G, Dejaco-Ruhswurm I, Funovics MA, et al. Outcome after treatment of ametropia with implantable contact lenses. Ophthalmology. 2003;**110**:2153-2161. DOI: 10.1016/S0161-6420(03)00830-3

[77] Güell JL, Morral M, Gris O, Gaytan J, Sisquella M, Manero F. Five-year follow-up of 399 phakic Artisan-Verisyse implantation for myopia, hyperopia, and/or astigmatism. Ophthalmology. 2008;**115**:1002-1012. DOI: 10.1016/j.ophtha.2007.08.022

[78] Chung JK, Lee SJ. Streptococcus mitis/oralis endophthalmitis management without phakic intraocular lens removal in patient with iris-fixated phakic intraocular lens implantation. BMC Ophthalmology. 2014;**14**:92. DOI: 10.1186/1471-2415-14-92

[79] Couto C, Rossetti S, Schlaen A, Hurtado E, D'Alessandro L, Goldstein DA. Chronic postoperative *Mycobacterium gordonae* endophthalmitis in a patient with phakic intraocular lens. Ocular Immunology and Inflammation. 2013;**21**:491-494. DOI: 10.3109/09273948.2013.824104

[80] Srinivasan B, Leung HY, Cao H, Liu S, Chen L, Fan AH. Modern phacoemulsification and intraocular lens implantation (refractive lens exchange) is safe and effective in treating high myopia. Asia-Pacific Journal of Ophthalmology. 2016;**5**:438-444. DOI: 10.1097/APO.0000000000000241

[81] Lundström M, Manning S, Barry P, Stenevi U, Henry Y, Rosen P. The European registry of quality outcomes for cataract and refractive surgery (EUREQUO): A database study of trends in volumes, surgical techniques and outcomes of refractive surgery. Eye Vision. 2015;**2**:8. DOI: 10.1186/s40662-015-0019-1

[82] Alio JL, Grzybowski A, El Aswad A, Romaniuk D. Refractive lens exchange. Survival Ophthalmology. Nov-Dec 2014;**59**(6):579-98. DOI: 10.1016/j.survophthal.2014.04.004. Epub 2014 May 9

[83] Braga-Mele R, Chang D, Dewey S, Foster G, Henderson BA, Hill W, et al. Multifocal intraocular lenses: Relative indications and contraindications for implantation. Journal of Cataract and Refractive Surgery. 2014;**40**:313-322. DOI: 10.1016/j.jcrs.2013.12.011

[84] Kamiya K, Hayashi K, Shimizu K, Negishi K, Sato M, Bissen-Miyajima H, et al. Multifocal intraocular lens explantation: A case series of 50 eyes. American Journal of Ophthalmology. 2014;**158**:215-220.e1. DOI: 10.1016/j.ajo.2014.04.010

[85] McNeely RN, Pazo E, Millar Z, Richoz O, Nesbit A, Moore TCB, et al. Threshold limit of postoperative astigmatism for patient satisfaction after refractive lens exchange and multifocal intraocular lens implantation. Journal of Cataract and Refractive Surgery. 2016;**42**:1126-1134. DOI: 10.1016/j.jcrs.2016.05.007

[86] Chong EW, Mehta JS. High myopia and cataract surgery. Current Opinion in Ophthalmology. 2016;**27**:45-50. DOI: 10.1097/ICU.0000000000000217

[87] Results of the Endophthalmitis Vitrectomy Study. A randomized trial of immediate vitrectomy and of intravenous antibiotics for the treatment of postoperative bacterial endophthalmitis. Endophthalmitis

Vitrectomy Study Group. Archives of Ophthalmology. 1995;**113**:1479-1496.

[88] Haigis W. Intraocular lens calculation in extreme myopia. Journal of Cataract and Refractive Surgery. 2009;**35**:906-911. DOI: 10.1016/j.jcrs.2008.12.035

[89] Yokoi T, Moriyama M, Hayashi K, Shimada N, Ohno-Matsui K. Evaluation of refractive error after cataract surgery in highly myopic eyes. International Ophthalmology. 2013;**33**:343-348. DOI: 10.1007/s10792-012-9690-6

[90] Fernández-Buenaga R, Alio JL, Pérez-Ardoy AL, Larrosa-Quesada A, Pinilla-Cortés L, Barraquer R, et al. Late in-the-bag intraocular lens dislocation requiring explantation: Risk factors and outcomes. Eye. 2013;**27**:795-801; quiz 802. DOI: 10.1038/eye.2013.95

[91] Soda M, Yaguchi S. Effect of decentration on the optical performance in multifocal intraocular lenses. Ophthalmologica. 2012;**227**:197-204. DOI: 10.1159/000333820

[92] Alio JL, Ruiz-Moreno JM, Shabayek MH, Lugo FL, Abd El Rahman AM, Alicante D. The risk of retinal detachment in high myopia after small incision coaxial phacoemulsification. American Journal of Ophthalmology. 2007;**144**:93-98. DOI: 10.1016/j.ajo.2007.03.043

[93] Vukicevic M, Gin T, Al-Qureshi S. Prevalence of optical coherence tomography-diagnosed postoperative cystoid macular oedema in patients following uncomplicated phaco-emulsification cataract surgery. Clinical & Experimental Ophthalmology. 2012;**40**:282-287. DOI: 10.1111/j.1442-9071.2011.02638.x

[94] Hayashi K, Ohno-Matsui K, Futagami S, Ohno S, Tokoro T, Mochizuki M. Choroidal neovascularization in highly myopic eyes after cataract surgery. Japanese Journal of Ophthalmology. 2006;**50**:345-348. DOI: 10.1007/s10384-006-0335-z

Section 5

Secondary Intraocular Lens Techniques

Chapter 9

Secondary Intraocular Lens

Niranjan Manoharan and Pradeep Prasad

Abstract

Secondary intraocular lens (IOL) implantation has evolved over the past few decades. Several new techniques, lens options, and materials now exist. Careful patient selection is important to determine the optimal secondary IOL technique. Intraocular lens placement in the capsular bag is the most ideal followed by sulcus placement. However, the best option when no capsular support exists in an aphakic patient remains unclear. Surgeons should be aware of contraindications for each technique; however, there are several situations where anterior chamber intraocular lens (ACIOL), scleral-fixated intraocular lens (SFIOL), and iris fixation can all be used. In those cases, surgeon familiarity and comfort with the secondary IOL technique can determine the type of surgery performed.

Keywords: secondary intraocular lens, aphakia, scleral fixated, iris fixated, anterior chamber intraocular lens

1. Introduction

Secondary intraocular lens implantation is defined as implantation of an intraocular lens following an initial surgery that resulted in aphakia or a deficient intraocular lens. The indications for secondary intraocular lens insertion have evolved with improved surgical outcomes of modern cataract surgery. Newer surgical techniques and lenses has also advanced the field of secondary intraocular lenses. The first wave of secondary intraocular lenses to be implanted was the anterior chamber intraocular lens (ACIOL) [1]. Secondary intraocular lenses can now be implanted in a variety of anatomic locations with different techniques used to support the lens (sutured, iris claw, etc.). Specifically, sutured IOL and intrascleral fixation techniques have been gaining popularity. Szigiato et al. found a 538% increase in secondary sutured IOL techniques from 2000 to 2013 [2]. However, with the advent of several new techniques there is no clear guidance for the best technique for secondary IOL placement. This chapter aims to discuss the variety of secondary intraocular lenses, the indications for use, and surgical considerations.

2. Indications

Modern cataract surgery has evolved the role of secondary intraocular lens implantation since there is now less incidence of surgical aphakia after cataract surgery [2]. With current technology and improved cataract surgery technique, the most common reason for secondary lens implantation is IOL exchange. The rates of IOL exchange also have declined over the years with recent studies showing rates of 0.34–0.77% [2–4]. ACIOL explantation is most commonly due to corneal decompensation and inflammation [5, 6]. PCIOL explantation is most commonly due to IOL decentration and dislocation [7]. IOL dislocation can be due to zonular dehiscence from trauma, previous complicated surgery, or conditions predisposing to zonular instability such as pseudoexfoliation syndrome and Marfan's syndrome.

Uveitis-hyphema-glaucoma (UGH) syndrome is a complication of iris chafing of an IOL. Most commonly this is due to a single-piece IOL with a haptic outside of the capsular bag that comes in contact with posterior iris tissue. IOL chafing of iris tissue leads to iris transillumination defects, pigment dispersion, microhyphema/hyphema, and glaucoma. Treatment of UGH often requires IOL removal with placement of a secondary IOL although in some cases the haptic in the sulcus alone can be cut and removed.

In recent years, advancements in IOL calculations, cataract surgery technology and technique have improved refractive outcomes. Patient visual expectations after cataract surgery have increased and now, in some cases, IOL exchanges are performed for unexpected refractive outcomes, dissatisfaction with multifocal lenses, and dysphotopsias following cataract surgery. The rates of IOL exchange due to patient dissatisfaction in one study showed an increase from 7.8% in 2005 to 21% in 2014 [3]. In 2005, no patients underwent IOL exchange for unsatisfactory refractive outcomes in the absence of optical aberrations but in 2014, 42% of IOL exchanges were due to unsatisfactory refractive outcomes alone.

3. Preoperative evaluation

Prior to consideration of secondary intraocular lens implantation, a thorough pre-operative history is required. In particular, details of the prior cataract removal including intraoperative complications, type of IOL implanted, location of the IOL implant and the presence of other ocular hardware including glaucoma drainage devices are important pieces of information to gather before secondary IOL surgery. To this end, review of prior operative reports and medical records is a critical element of every preoperative evaluation.

A thorough examination of the anterior and posterior segment is required to plan for a secondary IOL implantation. The conjunctiva and scleral should be examined to identify any prior incisional glaucoma surgery or devices. Corneal health should be evaluated to determine if an ACIOL is a viable option. Specular microscopy or pachymetry can be obtained as needed to assess corneal endothelial health. Anterior chamber depth should be evaluated as a narrow/shallow chamber might preclude safe ACIOL placement. The presence of vitreous prolapse in the anterior chamber should be noted as well as the integrity of the iris and capsule. Of note, high frequency ultrasound has shown to be better than slit lamp examination in assessing capsular support for sulcus IOL implantation [8]. If there is an intraocular lens in place, the type of lens and degree of dislocation should be assessed. The optic nerve and retina should be thoroughly examined to evaluate for any other ocular comorbidities that can limit vision potential or require treatment at the time of secondary IOL implantation. Finally, vision potential with a reliable manifest refraction is important to gauge the potential benefit of secondary IOL implantation.

4. Contact lens and aphakic glasses

Aphakic spectacles are a non-invasive option for bilateral aphakia although they are a sub-optimal solution for unilateral aphakia due to induced aniseikonia.

Aniseikonia is a significant difference in the perceived size of images between the two eyes. This difference in image sizes can be as large as 30% which makes fusion impossible [9]. Other drawbacks of aphakic spectacles are that they are heavy and have poor cosmesis since the lenses are thick centrally with significant magnification. Also, patients wearing aphakic lenses may notice a ring scotoma and have to cope with objects jumping in and out of their visual field.

Extended-wear contact lenses can be an adequate option for managing binocular and monocular aphakia. Properly fitted contact lenses can be well-tolerated by patients and secondary IOL implantation can be avoided in patients who are happy with contact lens use. Some physicians argue that a trial of aphakic contact lenses should be required prior to secondary IOL implantation, especially in eyes with questionable functional visual potential.

5. Determination of anatomic location of secondary IOL

Choosing the best location and technique for secondary IOL implantation can be a difficult one. No clear guidelines are established for secondary IOL implantation. In 2003, Wagoner et al. reviewed the literature on secondary IOL implantation [10]. In this paper, the authors found no evidence to claim superiority of any one technique or anatomic location for fixation. Since 2003, secondary IOL surgery has continued to evolve dramatically and still no clear evidence exists to guide surgeons. As Wagoner's paper noted, the most important factor often is the surgeon's comfort with a secondary IOL technique.

There are however, some recommendations in ruling out certain anatomic locations for IOL fixation. For example, poor corneal endothelial status and/or abnormal angle/iris anatomy should discourage anterior chamber IOL implantation. Lack of adequate iris support would rule out other iris-fixated approaches (sutured or iris-claw). Lack of posterior capsular support or a fibrosed anterior/posterior capsule would rule out in-the-bag PCIOL placement. Sulcus intraocular lens implantation requires adequate anterior capsular support. Scleral abnormalities (i.e., Marfan's, scleral thinning, etc.) would rule out scleral fixation techniques.

In-the-bag posterior chamber intraocular lens implantation remains the best anatomic location for an intraocular lens. However, even if during secondary IOL implantation the aphakic eye has an intact posterior capsule, the anterior/posterior capsule is typically fibrosed, preventing IOL implantation inside the capsular bag. Brunin et al. evaluated the complication rates, visual acuity and refractive outcomes of different intraocular lens implantation techniques [11]. Their study noted that capsular bag implantation had the best refractive outcomes followed by sulcus IOL with optic capture and sulcus IOL without optic capture. There was no difference between transscleral-sutured IOL, iris-fixated IOLs, and ACIOLs.

If possible, in-the-bag implantation has the best outcomes given its closest proximity to normal anatomy. This requires a stable and intact capsular bag. If no posterior capsular exists but there is adequate anterior capsular support, sulcus IOL implantation can be performed, preferably with optic capture. However, if no capsular support exists, the guidelines for secondary IOL implantation remain controversial [12]. If a viable 3-piece IOL has been dislocated, the preference might be to reposition the lens with an iris-sutured or scleral fixation technique. Other options include ACIOL implantation, iris-fixation techniques, and scleral-fixation techniques. The following sections will explore these options in more detail.

6. Capsular bag

Secondary intraocular lens implantation into the capsular bag can only be performed in the early post-operative period before the formation of anterior–posterior capsular adhesions. Typically, this procedure is performed in the early post-cataract surgery period due to incorrect intraocular lens power or patient dissatisfaction with an IOL (i.e., dysphotopsia from a multifocal IOL). Despite advances in IOL power formulas, some of which take into account the effects of prior refractive surgery, patients can still end up with large IOL power errors that may necessitate IOL exchange. Even with small errors, premium lens patients can demand IOL removal due to higher patient expectations in this population. IOL explantation in these cases should ideally be performed within 4–6 weeks of the initial cataract surgery although in-the-bag IOL exchange months to years following cataract surgery has been reported. A needle or cannula with viscoelastic is used to dissect the anterior capsular off the lens with care to avoid damaging zonular fibers and the posterior capsule. Once the lens is mobilized and removed, the capsular stability is assessed. If good anterior and posterior capsular support is noted the capsular bag is inflated with viscoelastic and a new lens can then be placed into the capsular bag.

7. Sulcus intraocular lens

Sulcus intraocular lens implantation is the second-best option if the anterior capsule is intact and in-the-bag implantation cannot be performed. In cases with a single-piece IOL dislocation, the IOL must be removed and replaced with a 3-piece IOL in the sulcus. In cases of 3-piece IOL dislocation, the IOL can be retrieved and repositioned into the ciliary sulcus. If the capsulorhexis is intact, the optic can then be captured by pushing the optic posteriorly through capsulorhexis with the lens haptics remaining in the sulcus. Of note, most three-piece IOLs have an overall haptic to haptic diameter of 13 mm or less, which can be too short especially in long eyes. This can lead to lens decentration and tilt. Three-piece intraocular lenses with larger haptics can fit better in the sulcus and decrease chances of decentration/tilt. With optic capture, the IOL calculations remain the same as the in-the-bag calculations [10].

Single-piece acrylic IOLs should not be placed in the sulcus [13–15]. Single-piece IOLs have haptics that are as thick as the optic and can chronically chafe the posterior iris causing uveitis-glaucoma-hyphema (UGH) syndrome. Unlike three-piece IOLs, which are posteriorly vaulted, single-piece IOLs are planar in configuration, increasing the potential contact between the optic and the iris. Furthermore, single piece IOLs are shorter in overall length than 3-piece IOLs and thus are not well supported in the sulcus leading to high rates of decentration and tilt.

7.1 Technique

Viscoelastic is used to create space between the iris and anterior capsular bag. The capsular bag should be evaluated to identify areas with optimal support. Iris mobilization with a Kuglen iris manipulator or expansion with iris hooks may be necessary for adequate visualization of the capsule. The haptics should be placed in areas where the anterior capsular support is greatest. The corneal incision should be planned along the axis where IOL haptic placement is desired. The lens is then inserted with the leading haptic inserted on top of the anterior capsular bag and underneath the iris. However, if the corneal incision is not in the axis of desired haptic placement the lens can be inserted with the haptics on top of the iris. The lens is than rotated to the desired axis on top of the iris. Once in the desired axis the haptics are then placed into the sulcus. The trailing haptic is then rotated into the sulcus with a second instrument. The intraocular lens is then checked for stability and centration. If possible, the optic can be captured into the anterior capsule. There is no indication for peripheral iridotomy with sulcus intraocular lens implantation.

8. Iris-fixated intraocular lens

A secondary IOL can be fixated to iris tissue by suture or iris-claw enclavation. Iris-fixated secondary IOLs have the benefit of sparing scleral/conjunctival surgery in case future glaucoma surgery is needed, however normal iris anatomy is required. Iris fixation can cause iris chafing leading to inflammation and cystoid macular edema. As with all secondary IOL techniques, patient selection and counseling are key for surgical success.

A three-piece IOL can also be sutured to the iris via a variety of techniques. In one technique, the IOL is inserted into the anterior chamber such that the optic is captured by the iris with the haptics located behind the iris. A 10-0 prolene suture on a long-curved needle is used to suture the haptic to the iris with as small a bite as possible and placed as peripherally as possible. Peripheral placement avoids creating an oval iris. The suture is then tied in place and the ends trimmed. A smaller corneal incision can be used as the IOLs for this technique are foldable.

Iris-claw lenses are the most commonly used iris-fixation technique outside of the United States. Several studies have shown the safety and efficacy of this technique [16, 17]. A peripheral iridectomy is required to decrease the risk of pupillary block. Iris-claw lenses need to be carefully centered during enclavation. Studies have shown that if the iris-claw lens undergoes deenclavation, the haptics are irreversibly damaged, and the lens requires explanation [18]. These lenses can be fixated anterior or posterior to the iris. A 5-year follow-up showed no differences in astigmatism, complications or post-operative corneal endothelial cell density between anterior or posterior placement [19]. However, some prefer posterior placement with the theory that deenclavation posteriorly has less risk of corneal endothelial decompensation compared to the anterior approach [20].

9. Scleral-fixated intraocular lens

Scleral-fixated intraocular lenses have gained popularity for secondary IOL implantation in patients with aphakia. They are indicated in patients who do not wish to remain aphakic and have no capsular or iris support. However, some surgeons prefer SFIOLs even if there is iris support. In patients where an ACIOL might not be a good option such as in patients with corneal endothelial disease or glaucoma, SFIOLs or IFIOLs are both viable options.

Scleral-sutured intraocular lens implantation started in the 1980s with ab-interno and ab-externo approaches. Ab-interno approaches utilized suture passes from inside to outside the eye in a blind maneuver. This led to complications with retinal detachment, vitreous hemorrhage, and unpredictable haptic placement. Ab-externo approaches were found to be more promising with sutures passed from outside to inside the eye. This led to more reliable suture placement. Lewis popularized an ab-externo technique in 1991 [21] whereby 10-0 polypropylene suture was placed 2 mm posterior to the limbus and then "docked" into a 28-gauge straight needle 180 degrees away to externalize the needle. The suture that remained inside the eye was brought out through the corneal incision and cut. The suture ends were then tied to the IOL haptics and the IOL was inserted into the eye for sulcus placement. The external sutures were then tied down to the adjacent sclera. Ten-year follow-up of thirteen eyes showed only two eyes had minimal decentration although it did not affect final visual acuity [22].

Since Lewis described his technique, newer lenses and sutures have further improved ab-externo techniques. Lenses such as the CZ70BD (Alcon, Fort Worth, TX), enVista MX60 and the Akreos AO60 (Bausch and Lomb, Rochester, NY) have eyelets for suture fixation, which improve lens stability. Most prior scleral suture-fixed techniques used 10-0 polypropylene. However, several studies have described 10-0 polypropylene late suture breakage [23–25]. These reports show late breakage of 10-0 polypropylene suture up to 8 years post-placement. Gore-tex sutures have been used outside the eye with notable long-term stability. Studies with up to 3 years follow-up have shown Gore-tex suture durability within the eye. Similarly, 9-0 polypropylene has been shown to have improved suture stability compared to 10-0 polypropylene but with only short-term follow-up. Long-term studies are needed to further evaluate if these sutures continue to avoid suture breakage.

Bausch & Lomb Akreos AO60 hydrophilic acrylic lens contains 4 eyelets allowing 4 point fixation. However, these lenses undergo calcification and opacify when in contact with intraocular gas or air [26]. Given that aphakic patients often have coincident retinal pathology and might be at increased risk for retinal detachment repair this might be an important consideration when deciding on the optimal lens and fixation technique. The Bausch & Lomb enVista Mx60 IOL is made of hydrophobic acrylic and does not opacify when in contact with gas or air. However, it has only 2 eyelets for fixation at the haptic-optic junction.

9.1 Scleral fixation of IOL with Gore-tex suture technique

Typically, conjunctival peritomies are performed where the sclerotomy sites are planned, 180 degrees apart. Sclerotomy placement at horizontal, oblique and vertical orientations are all acceptable. A toric lens marker is used to mark the axis of the lens within the peritomy. Sclerotomy sites are marked, 3 mm posterior to the limbus and 4–5 mm apart from each other in each scleral bed. One of the suture sclerotomy sites can be used for the vitrectomy trocar. The trocar sclerotomy should be made perpendicularly without tunneling to facilitate suture knot insertion. The lens is pre-threaded with a suture on each side and inserted into the eye. The sutures are then externalized using forceps through the sclerotomies taking care not to tangle the sutures. To avoid suture tangling and disorganization, the sutures can be inserted into the eye and externalized prior to lens insertion. The sutures are then tied down permanently with care taken to make sure the suture tension allows the lens to be appropriately centered. The knot is then buried into the sclerotomies to avoid knot erosion through the conjunctiva. The conjunctiva is sewn in place over the sclerotomies and sutured. Long term follow-up results are yet to be determined. Two-year results have shown good lens and suture stability with the Gore-tex suture. Complications include hypotony (up to 10%) with and without serous choroidal detachment. This is thought to occur from leakage from the sclerotomy sites. Vitreous hemorrhage and hyphema have also been reported. Published studies have not reported persistent post-operative inflammation, endophthalmitis or suture erosion/breakage at 2 years [27]. With in-the-bag calculations for the IOL, a recent study showed that 2 mm sclerotomies resulted in a more myopic post-operative outcome than 3 mm sclerotomies [28]. Other studies have shown acceptable refractive outcomes with this technique and 3 mm from the limbus sclerotomies with in-the-bag IOL calculations [29].

9.2 Sutureless scleral fixation intraocular lens implantation

Sutureless techniques have also been developed to avoid potential complications that can rise from suture fixation including knot erosion, endophthalmitis, and suture breakage. Agarwal described scleral fixation with glued haptic fixation [30]. Scleral flaps are created 180 degrees apart and a sclerotomy is made within the flap. The haptics of a 3-piece IOL are then externalized via the sclerotomy and glued into place with the flap closing over the haptic. Several complications can occur with the haptic including extrusion, dislocation, and breakage. Haptic-related complications seen include haptic extrusion, haptic dislodgement, broken haptic and subconjunctival haptic. Most of the haptic-related complications are due to improper scleral tucking [31].

Yamane et al. described a technique whereby three-piece IOL haptics are passed through a 27 gauge needle which guides the haptic through a tunneled sclerotomy [32]. The externalized haptic is than cauterized to create a bulb at the tip of the haptic to allow for improved stability within the scleral tunnel. Short-term outcomes from Yamane's initial study reported no IOL dislocation at 1.5 years. Reported complications include optic capture of the iris (8%), vitreous hemorrhage (5%) and cystoid macular edema (1%). It is important to note that the Yamane technique utilizes the EC-3 PAL three-piece intraocular lens, which has more durable and malleable haptics compared to the 3-piece IOLs commonly used in the United States. Higher rates of IOL dislocation have been reported with the Yamane technique when non-EC-3 PAL 3-piece IOLs are used. Several modified Yamane techniques have been since described including the use of 27 gauge trocars instead of a needle to externalize the haptics. Long-term follow-up has yet to be presented since these techniques have only been introduced in the past decade.

10. Anterior chamber intraocular lens

Baron was the first to implant an anterior chamber IOL in 1952 [33]. Several other ACIOLs followed during the 1950s but were limited by their design and anterior vault that led to high rates of corneal decompensation. Closed loop ACIOLs gained popularity in the 1970s due to their various flexible designs that were thought to alleviate problems with sizing. However, the sharp edges of the closed-loop ACIOL haptic eroded uveal tissue, released inflammatory mediators, and led to multiple complications including uveitis-glaucoma-hyphema syndrome, corneal decompensation, and cystoid macular edema [34–37]. Open-loop ACIOL designs were introduced in the 1980s and their design continued to be improved with its use peaking in the 1990s. These modern open-loop ACIOL designs appear to have less associated complications.

A peripheral iridectomy is required as ACIOLs can cause pupillary block glaucoma. Compared to other IOL techniques, the ACIOL requires a larger six-millimeter incision. Typically, a scleral tunnel is formed in order to minimize astigmatism from a clear corneal incision. Contraindications for anterior chamber intraocular lens include corneal decompensation, angle abnormalities with or without glaucoma, and lack of iris support. Complications associated with ACIOL implantation include endothelial failure with corneal edema, chronic intraocular inflammation, and/or uveitis glaucoma hyphema. The angle to angle measurement measured by a UBM or OCT is the most accurate option for fitting an ACIOL. More commonly however the white-to-white distance is measured intraoperatively with calipers and 1 mm is added to size the ACIOL. The white-to-white distance is not always a reliable equivalent to the actual angle to angle distance.

Many of the complications of ACIOL implantation can be prevented with an appropriately-sized lens, however, limited sizes are available. An overly small lens can be mobile and cause damage to the corneal endothelium leading to corneal decompensation. A small lens can also cause trauma to iris tissue leading to inflammation and cystoid macular edema. Similarly, an overly large lens can cause inflammation, cystoid macular edema and corneal endothelial failure. A large lens can be noted if the iris is distorted or ovalized during placement. This is due to the footplates not being seated well in the angle. Since the vertical and horizontal angle to angle dimensions are different the lens can be rotated to see if it fits better at a different meridian.

10.1 Anterior chamber intraocular lens implantation technique

A scleral tunnel is created in either a frown or linear configuration. This can be placed temporally or superiorly based on surgeon preference. A corneal incision is avoided to minimize astigmatism however can be used if needed. The benefits of a corneal incision include preserving conjunctiva/sclera for potential glaucoma interventions. Miosis is induced and viscoelastic is then injected. The ACIOL is then inserted with or without a use of a lens glide. The purpose of the lens glide to secure placement of the ACIOL across the pupil so as not to get the lens or haptic caught on the iris at the pupillary margin. The ACIOL is then positioned such that the footplates of the IOL are well-seated in the angle and the pupillary margin is round. Gonioscopy can be performed to confirm appropriate placement of the ACIOL footplates. Once the ACIOL is positioned, a peripheral iridectomy is created and the scleral or corneal incision is closed.

11. Conclusion

Ophthalmology has seen an evolution in secondary intraocular lens implantation. Particularly, in the past decade, the implantation of scleral-fixated intraocular lenses has gained popularity along with ACIOL implantation [36]. Careful patient selection is critical to determine the optimal secondary IOL technique. When possible, placement of the secondary intraocular lens in the capsular bag is preferred, followed by placement in the sulcus with optic capture. When capsular support is absent, ACIOL implantation, iris fixation and scleral fixation of a secondary intraocular lens can be considered. The variety of surgical options with respect to secondary IOL implantation illustrates the lack of an optimal consensus technique. Indeed, several studies have compared these techniques with no clear favorite [38–41]. In most cases, patient ophthalmic history and anatomic considerations in addition to surgeon familiarity and comfort with the secondary IOL technique may determine the type of surgery performed.

Secondary Intraocular Lens
DOI: http://dx.doi.org/10.5772/intechopen.89569

Author details

Niranjan Manoharan and Pradeep Prasad*
Stein Eye Institute, University of California, Los Angeles, CA, United States

*Address all correspondence to: prasad@jsei.ucla.edu

IntechOpen

© 2019 The Author(s). Licensee IntechOpen. This chapter is distributed under the terms of the Creative Commons Attribution License (http://creativecommons.org/licenses/by/3.0), which permits unrestricted use, distribution, and reproduction in any medium, provided the original work is properly cited. (cc) BY

References

[1] Rattigan SM et al. Flexible open-loop anterior chamber intraocular lens implantation after posterior capsule complications in extracapsular cataract extraction. Journal of Cataract & Refractive Surgery. 1996;**22**(2):243-246

[2] Szigiato A-A, Schlenker MB, Ahmed IIK. Population-based analysis of intraocular lens exchange and repositioning. Journal of Cataract & Refractive Surgery. 2017;**43**(6):754-760

[3] Jones JJ, Jones YJ, Jin GJC. Indications and outcomes of intraocular lens exchange during a recent 5-year period. American Journal of Ophthalmology. 2014;**157**(1):154-162

[4] Jin GJC, Crandall AS, Jones JJ. Changing indications for and improving outcomes of intraocular lens exchange. American Journal of Ophthalmology. 2005;**140**(4):688-694

[5] Solomon KD et al. Complications of intraocular lenses with special reference to an analysis of 2500 explanted intraocular lenses (IOLs). European Journal of Implant and Refractive Surgery. 1991;**3**(3):195-200

[6] Marques FF et al. Longitudinal study of intraocular lens exchange. Journal of Cataract & Refractive Surgery. 2007;**33**(2):254-257

[7] Leysen I et al. Surgical outcomes of intraocular lens exchange: Five-year study. Journal of Cataract & Refractive Surgery. 2009;**35**(6):1013-1018

[8] De Silva DJ, Nischal KK, Packard RB. Preoperative assessment of secondary intraocular lens implantation for aphakia: A comparison of 2 techniques. Journal of Cataract & Refractive Surgery. 2005;**31**(7):1351-1356

[9] Repka MX. Visual rehabilitation in pediatric aphakia. Pediatric Cataract. 2016;**57**:49-68

[10] Wagner M, Cox T, Ariyasu R. Intraocular lens implantation in absence of capsular support. Ophthalmology. 2003;**110**:840-859

[11] Brunin G et al. Secondary intraocular lens implantation: Complication rates, visual acuity, and refractive outcomes. Journal of Cataract & Refractive Surgery. 2017;**43**(3):369-376

[12] Dalby M, Kristianslund O, Drolsum L. Long-term outcomes after surgery of late in-the-bag intraocular lens dislocation: A randomized clinical trial. American Journal of Ophthalmology. 2019;**207**:184-194

[13] Kemp PS, Oetting TA. Stability and safety of MA50 intraocular lens placed in the sulcus. Eye (London, England). 2015;**29**(11):1438-1441

[14] Chang DF, Masket S, Miller KM, Braga-Mele R, Little BC, Mamalis N, et al. Complications of sulcus placement of single-piece acrylic intraocular lenses recommendations for backup IOL implantation following posterior capsule rupture. Journal of Cataract and Refractive Surgery. 2009;**35**(8):1445-1458

[15] Mohebbi M, Bashiri SA, Mohammadi SF, Samet B, Ghassemi F, Ashrafi E, et al. Outcome of single-piece intraocular lens sulcus implantation following posterior capsular rupture during phacoemulsification. Journal of Ophthalmic & Vision Research. 2017;**12**(3):275-280

[16] Anbari A, Lake DB. Posteriorly enclavated iris claw intraocular lens for aphakia: Long-term corneal endothelial

safety study. European Journal of Ophthalmology. 2015;**25**(3):208-213

[17] Schallenberg M et al. Aphakia correction with retropupillary fixated iris-claw lens (Artisan)—Long-term results. Clinical Ophthalmology (Auckland, NZ). 2014;**8**:137

[18] Tandogan T et al. Material analysis of spontaneously subluxated iris-fixated phakic intraocular lenses. Journal of Refractive Surgery. 2016;**32**(9):618-625

[19] Toro MD et al. Five-year follow-up of secondary iris-claw intraocular lens implantation for the treatment of aphakia: Anterior chamber versus retropupillary implantation. PloS one. 2019;**14**(4):e0214140

[20] Lajoie J et al. Assessment of astigmatism associated with the iris-fixated ARTISAN aphakia implant: Anterior fixation versus posterior fixation, study of postoperative follow-up at one year. Journal Francais D'Ophtalmologie. 2018;**41**(8):696-707

[21] Lewis JS. Ab externo sulcus fixation. Ophthalmic Surgery. 1991;**22**(11):692-695

[22] Cavallini GM, Volante V, De Maria M, et al. Long-term analysis of IOL stability of the Lewis technique for scleral fixation. European Journal of Ophthalmology. 2015;**25**(6):525-528

[23] Assia EI, Nemet A, Sachs D. Bilateral spontaneous subluxation of scleral-fixated intraocular lenses. Journal of Cataract and Refractive Surgery. 2002;**28**(12):2214-2216

[24] Bading G, Hillenkamp J, Sachs HG, Gabel VP, Framme C. Long-term safety and functional outcome of combined pars plana vitrectomy and scleral-fixated sutured posterior chamber lens implantation. American Journal of Ophthalmology. 2007;**144**(3):371-377

[25] Malta JB, Banitt M, Musch DC, Sugar A, Mian SI, Soong HK. Long-term outcome of combined penetrating keratoplasty with scleral-sutured posterior chamber intraocular lens implantation. Cornea. 2009;**28**(7):741-746

[26] Kalevar A, Dollin M, Gupta RR. Opacification of scleral-sutured akreos AO60 intraocular lens after vitrectomy with gas tamponade: Case series. Retinal Cases & Brief Reports. 2017:1-4

[27] Khan MA et al. Scleral fixation of intraocular lenses using Gore-Tex suture: Clinical outcomes and safety profile. British Journal of Ophthalmology. 2016;**100**(5):638-643

[28] Su D et al. Refractive outcomes after pars plana vitrectomy and scleral fixated intraocular lens with gore-tex suture. Ophthalmology Retina. Jul 2019;**3**(7):548-552

[29] Botsford BW et al. Scleral fixation of intraocular lenses with Gore-Tex suture: Refractive outcomes and comparison of lens power formulas. Ophthalmology Retina. Jun 2019;**3**(6):468-472

[30] Narang P, Narang S. Glue-assisted intrascleral fixation of posterior chamber intraocular lens. Indian Journal of Ophthalmology. 2013;**61**(4):163

[31] Kumar DA, Agarwal A. Glued intraocular lens: A major review on surgical technique and results. Current Opinion in Ophthalmology. 2013;**24**(1):21-29

[32] Yamane S, Inoue M, Arakawa A, Kadonosono K. Sutureless 27-gauge needle-guided intrascleral intraocular lens implantation with lamellar scleral dissection. Ophthalmology. 2014;**121**(1):61-66

[33] Anterior chamber intraocular lenses. Survey of Ophthalmology. 2000;**45**:S131-S149

[34] Apple DJ et al. Anterior chamber lenses. Part II: A laboratory study. Journal of Cataract & Refractive Surgery. 1987;**13**(2):175-189

[35] Apple DJ et al. Anterior chamber lenses. Part I: Complications and pathology and a review of designs. Journal of Cataract & Refractive Surgery. 1987;**13**(2):157-174

[36] Apple DJ, Olson RJ. Closed-loop anterior chamber lenses. Archives of Ophthalmology. 1987;**105**(1):19-20

[37] Apple DH et al. Intraocular lenses: Evolution, Designs, Complications, and Pathology. Archives of Ophthalmology. 1991;**109**(2):189

[38] Madhivanan N et al. Comparative analysis of retropupillary iris claw versus scleral-fixated intraocular lens in the management of post-cataract aphakia. Indian Journal of Ophthalmology. 2019;**67**(1):59

[39] Nehme J et al. Secondary intraocular lens implantation with absence of capsular support: Scleral versus iris fixation. Journal Francais D'Ophtalmologie. 2018;**41**(7):630-636

[40] Kim EJ, Brunin GM, Al-Mohtaseb ZN. Lens placement in the absence of capsular support: Scleral-fixated versus iris-fixated IOL versus ACIOL. International Ophthalmology Clinics. 2016;**56**(3):93-106

[41] Kim KH, Kim WS. Comparison of clinical outcomes of iris fixation and scleral fixation as treatment for intraocular lens dislocation. American Journal of Ophthalmology. 2015;**160**(3):463-469

Chapter 10

Scleral-Fixated Intraocular Lens: Indications and Results

Simona-Delia Nicoară

Abstract

Currently, ideal cataract surgery should end with the placement of an intraocular lens (IOLs) in the bag. However, in the clinical setting we have to manage cases without enough capsular support to allow the physiological IOL placement. Progress has been made in terms of IOL designs and implantation techniques. The options should be analyzed not only in accordance with surgeon's experience but also with patient's age, local, and systemic comorbidities. Thus, in the absence of an appropriate capsule, IOL can be placed in the anterior chamber, fixated to the iris or to the sclera wall. In this paper, the personal experience of one surgeon with ab externo scleral-fixated IOLs is presented, with the aim to outline the place of this surgical technique in the correction of aphakia. A retrospective study was carried out, including 57 patients in which an IOL was fixated to the sclera, throughout January 2015–April 2019. The causes of aphakia, preoperative and postoperative best-corrected visual acuities (BCVA), and intra- and postoperative complications are analyzed. Statistical tests were applied in order to draw significance. In most instances, BCVA has remained stable, with no significant complications, making sclera fixation IOL a viable solution in the correction of aphakia.

Keywords: scleral-fixated IOL, aphakia, cataract surgery, eye trauma, lens dislocation

1. Introduction

Ideal correction of aphakia means the placement of the intraocular lens (IOLs) in the bag which relies on good capsular support [1–3]. In these circumstances, IOL is well centered to the pupillary axis, maximizing the chances of optimal surgical and refractive outcomes [2].

In the absence of adequate posterior capsular support, like in complicated cataract surgery with disruption of the posterior capsule, it is often possible to place the IOL in the sulcus with excellent visual outcome [1, 3].

However, in the clinical practice there are situations like trauma, diseases, and complicated cataract surgery that result in inadequate anterior and posterior capsular support, making the conventional in-the-bag or in the sulcus placement of the IOL impossible.

Addressing this situation can be managed in several ways, like anterior chamber (ACIOLs), iris-fixated (IFIOLs), and scleral-fixated (SFIOLs) [2, 3]. Choosing the best technique in the absence of capsular support can be challenging, although all these variants proved to have similar benefits and risks [2, 3].

A vitreoretinal surgeon is relatively frequently confronted with the situation to place an IOL in an eye without capsular support following the various conditions: trauma, complicated cataract surgery, and different ocular diseases. Trauma is of special interest, since it affects younger patients and is frequently followed by other changes in eye anatomy that add difficulty to the IOL implantation procedure. General conditions such as Marfan syndrome and homocystinuria affect young people with long life expectancy, so finding the best long-term solution for them is mandatory.

After an overview on the possibilities to correct aphakia in the absence of capsular support, with focus on the SFIOLs, personal experience with SFIOLs will be presented.

2. Correction of aphakia in the absence of capsular support: Overview

When facing an aphakic eye with no capsular support, the IOL can be placed in the anterior chamber, fixated to the iris (in its extreme or mid-periphery) or fixated to the sclera. The surgical techniques in all of these approaches have improved considerably over the last decades with subsequent optimization of visual and ocular outcomes [3].

2.1 ACIOLs

Placement of an IOL in the AC requires a healthy endothelium and a normal depth of the AC [2]. This technique has the advantages of being simple and quick. Modern designs of ACIOLs with flexible open-loop haptics and anteriorly vaulted optics make them beneficial for many patients [2]. However, they are not suitable for patients with glaucoma, endothelial compromise, significant iris trauma, or diabetic retinopathy.

Complications related to ACIOLs, even if rarer now, are still cited: uveitis-glaucoma-hyphema (UGH) syndrome and cystoid macular edema [2]. The general idea is that ACIOLs are in decline, as their placement requires bigger incisions, more astigmatism with suturing, and slower visual recovery [2].

2.2 IFIOLs

Some surgeons' experience reveals that IFIOLs are more efficient than ACIOLs and even developed an ideal patient profile benefiting from them: older, with average-sized anterior segments, especially if they have some remnants of capsule and vitreous that help stabilize the lens. The haptics have to be fixated to the iris as peripherally as possible. The complications associated with this type of implant are intra- and postoperative hyphema, cystoid macular edema, uveitis, and glaucoma. Even if the IFIOL is properly fixated, there is a certain degree of IOL mobility, with subsequent mechanical trauma from pseudophacodonesis, which is why most surgeons do not indicate them in younger patients [2]. Another reason of concern is suture longevity, requiring another surgery down the road [2].

The sutureless iris-claw IOLs are inserted through a 5-mm incision and are attached to the mid-peripheral iris with the help of an inclavation needle that grabs iris tissue between claws on either side of the lens while the pupil is kept miotic. A study of 2 years follow-up showed good visual functional recovery and lack of complications related to this technique [2].

2.3 SFIOLs

An IOL can be fixated at the sclera in several ways: with sutures, with no sutures by tunneling of the haptics, and with fibrin glue.

Suturing an IOL to the sclera is the most technically demanding procedure among the others discussed here, but it has two major advantages: durability and security.

When dealing with a dislocated IOL, several factors have to be considered: IOL type, extent of dislocation, and status of the capsular bag. If a one-piece in the bag IOL is partially dislocated, trans-scleral suture fixation is preferred. If a one-piece IOL is completely dislocated, it is recommended to be replaced with a three-piece IOL which is sutured to the sclera. If retinal pathology is associated, it is preferable to leave the eye aphakic to quiet down and perform the implantation in a second step. For example, once the retinal detachment is fixed and stable, a scleral-fixated three-piece IOL is carried out.

SFIOLs have drawbacks too. The patient is left with a subconjunctival suture, so in case of conjunctival erosion, the suture is exposed and makes way for bacteria to enter the eye and cause endophthalmitis. Therefore, it is desirable to bury the sutures. In order to prevent conjunctival erosion, Lewis imagined a method to bury the knot under a triangular scleral flap performed before entering the eye and the covering of the knot with the hinged scleral tissue at the end of surgery [3].

To avoid the use of sutures, tunneling of IOL haptics was imagined [2].

Another method to secure the IOL at the sclera is with fibrin glue. The pioneer of this technique advocates that it inhibits pseudophacodonesis better than the other variants. IOL movement inside the eye generates inflammation which is at the origin of cystoid macular edema [2].

An issue related to IOL fixation at the sclera comes from the fact that surgery is performed at pars plana, which is a region where anterior segment surgeon does not feel very comfortable. This is why this technique is preferred mostly by vitreoretinal surgeons.

All of the abovementioned alternatives to fixate an IOL inside an aphakic eye without capsular support produce good visual outcomes. Decision-making process relies on several factors: eye anatomy, other pathologies, patient's age, visual potential, and surgeon's comfort. It is equally important to know when a certain technique is contraindicated. Ideally, ophthalmic surgeon should master several techniques and be able to adjust plans during surgery [2].

3. Scleral-fixated intraocular lens: Indications and results: Personal experience

3.1 Aim

In this paper, the personal experience of one surgeon with ab interno scleral-fixated IOLs is presented, with the aim to outline the place of this surgical technique in the correction of aphakia.

3.2 Methods

This is a retrospective study that includes 57 aphakic eyes belonging to 57 patients who underwent ab interno scleral fixation of IOL during January 2015 to April 2019 at our tertiary care Ophthalmological Department, Emergency County Hospital from Cluj-Napoca, Romania. The patients were in the 10–89 years age group.

The detailed history was taken from each patient regarding any systemic or ocular condition. A written informed consent was taken from each patient before procedure.

Ophthalmological examination included grading of the visual acuity (VA) with the decimal system, followed by slit lamp examination of the anterior and posterior segment, examination of retinal periphery, and measurement of intraocular pressure by applanation tonometry. B-scan and OCT were performed whenever necessary. A-scan biometry was carried out before the procedure in all cases to find the value of the IOL to be implanted.

The data were analyzed statistically with the Program SPSS 21.0. Chi-square test was used to find statistical significance. A p-value ˂ 0.05 was considered significant.

This study was approved by the Ethics Committee belonging to the "Iuliu Hatieganu" University of Medicine and Pharmacy, and it is performed in accordance with the Declaration of Helsinki regarding the clinical studies involving human subjects.

3.3 Surgical procedure

All patients were operated by the same surgeon in local anesthesia, with the exception of one 10-year-old child with Marfan syndrome.

Pars plana vitrectomy (PPV) was performed in all cases to remove the lens/nucleus/IOL from the vitreous. The three subluxated lenses were removed by pars plana approach (lensectomy).

Conjunctival peritomies were created superiorly, then at horizontal meridians. Triangular partial-thickness (about 1/3 of the scleral thickness) limbal-based scleral flaps were dissected at horizontal meridians (9 o'clock and 3 o'clock position).

Intraocular pressure (IOP) was maintained with pars plana scleral infusion throughout surgery.

A 6-mm sclerocorneal tunnel incision was created superiorly, at 12 o'clock position, and anterior chamber (AC) was entered with a 2.2-mm knife. All vitreous was removed from the anterior chamber, if present, with the posterior vitrector. In the meantime, the two sutures (10–0 PC9 polypropylene) had been fixed to the IOL haptics of the specially designed IOL (**Figure 1**).

The long-curved needle carrying the 10–0 PC9 suture entered the AC and then exteriorized through the sclera, at 9 o'clock meridian, about 1–2 mm posterior from the posterior surgical limbus. The procedure was repeated similarly with the second needle (**Figure 2**).

The IOL was inserted in the sulcus, while the sutures were pulled, in order to center it. The haptics were secured at the sclera with knots that were buried under the previously fashioned scleral flaps (**Figure 3**).

Corneoscleral incision was sutured with 10–0 polypropylene sutures and the conjunctiva, with 8–0 vicryl sutures (**Figure 4**).

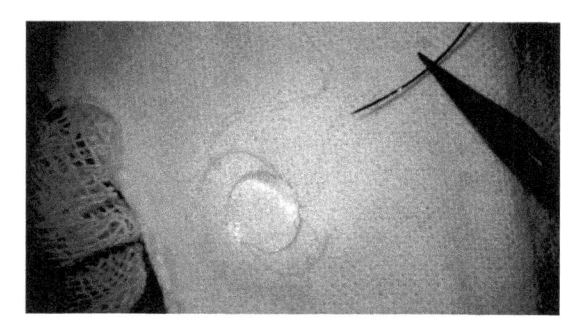

Figure 1.
IOL for scleral fixation - model CZ 70 BD (Alcon).

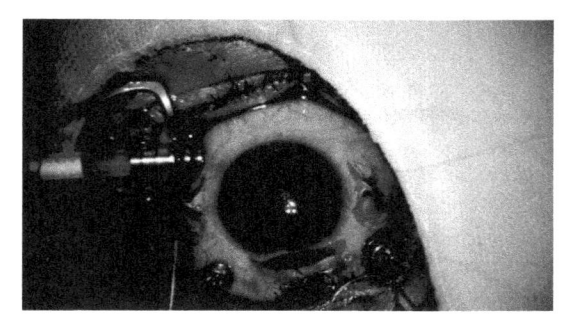

Figure 2.
Ab interno IOL implantation by suturing it to the sclera. Scleral flaps are visible at the horizontal meridian.

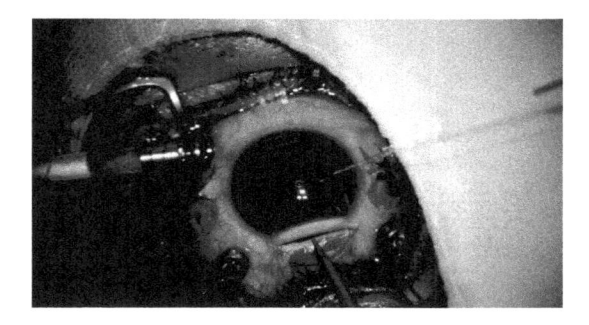

Figure 3.
IOL is pushed behind the iris, whereas the 2 sutures are pulled in order to center it.

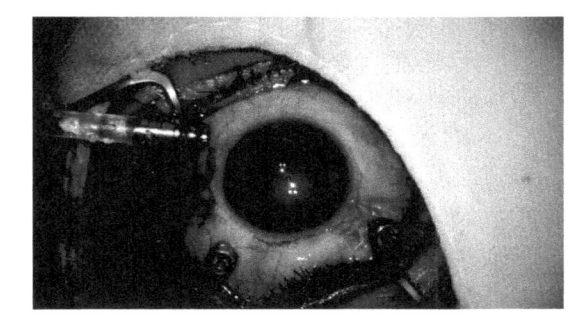

Figure 4.
IOL is well centered, the conjunctiva is sutured, the 3 ports of PPV are visible.

All patients were examined the next day after surgery, followed 1 week and then every month, for 3 months. At each visit, best-corrected visual acuity (BCVA) was noted and slit lamp examination, indirect ophthalmoscopy, and IOP measurement were performed. Wherever necessary, ultrasound and OCT examination were carried out.

In all cases, CZ70BD (Alcon, Fort Worth, TX) has been used. It incorporates eyelets on each haptic through which sutures can be passed that help to prevent suture slippage and subsequent IOL dislocation. Since this IOL has only two eyelets, two-point fixation technique has been used in all cases. The suture of choice was 10–0 polypropylene with PC9 needles.

3.4 Results

Fifty-seven patients were included in this study, with a mean age of 64.22 years. Minimum age in our series was 10 years, whereas maximum age was 89 years. Age distribution of patients is presented in **Table 1**.

Out of 57 patients, 40 were males (70.17%) and 17 were females (29.82%).

The cause that led to aphakia requiring scleral fixation of the IOL was represented by trauma in 30 patients (52.63%), complicated cataract surgery in 24 patients (42.10%), and subluxated lens in 3 patients (5.26%).

Medium age within the three groups was 61.10 years within the trauma group, 65.20 years within the postcataract surgery group, and 37 years within the subluxated lens group. These data are summarized in **Table 2**.

Within the trauma group, 24 patients were males (80%) and 6 patients were females (20%). Within the complicated cataract surgery group, 15 patients were males (62.50%) and 9 were females (37.50%). Within the subluxated lens group, one patient was male (33.33%) and two were females (66.66%).

T-test found a p-value <0.05 when comparing gender distribution between the first two groups: there was significantly more men than women within the trauma group as opposed to the postcataract surgery group.

Preoperative BCVA ranged between hand motion (HM) and 5/10, and it is illustrated in **Table 3**.

Preoperative BCVA according to the cause is illustrated in **Table 4**.

In nine cases (15.78%), there was a history of retinal detachment (RD) prior to IOL suture: five within the group of patients with complicated cataract surgery and four within the trauma group. In these circumstances, the strategy was to operate first RD, and if the retina was stable after tamponade agent removal, scleral fixation of the IOL was performed.

In five cases from the trauma group, an IOL was luxated into the vitreous cavity. In all situations we replaced it with an IOL specially designed for scleral fixation: CZ70BD (Alcon, Fort Worth, TX).

In six cases from the trauma group, an intraocular foreign body had been removed by PPV several months prior to IOL fixation.

Age decade	Number of patients	%
<50	12	21.05
51–60	8	14.03
61–70	10	17.54
71–80	19	33.33
>80	8	14.03

Table 1.
Age distribution of patients with scleral-fixated IOL.

Cause	Number of cases	%	Medium age (years)
Trauma	30	52.63	61.10
Postcataract	24	42.10	65.20
Surgery Subluxated lens	3	5.26	37

Table 2.
Causes of aphakia and medium age according to it.

BCVA	Before surgery (%)	Last visit after surgery (%)
‹1/50	7 (12.28)	4 (7.01)
≥1/50 ‹1/10	32 (56.14)	28 (56.14)
≥1/10	18 (31.57)	25 (43.85)

Table 3.
BCVA before and at the last visit after surgery.

Cause/BCVA	‹1/50	≥1/50 ‹1/10	≥1/10
Trauma	4	13	13
Previous cataract	3	16	5
Surgery subluxated lens	—	3	—

Table 4.
Preoperative BCVA according to the cause.

In two cases we noted breaking of sutures during surgery which was solved by replacing it. Breakage of one IOL haptic was encountered in one case, and it was solved by IOL replacement.

Intraoperatively soft eye was encountered in 11 cases (19.29%), and it was solved by adjusting the infusion pressure.

The most common complication during surgery was hemorrhage: 20/57 cases (35.08%). It was mild/moderate, and self-limiting, and it happened during puncturing the sclera with the PC9 needle in all cases. The blood was washed out with the PPV infusion system.

In the postoperative period, vitreous hemorrhage persisted in 10 cases (17.54%) and resolved spontaneously in 9 of them. PPV was performed in the remaining case, 4 weeks after IOL fixation, with good outcome: BCVA 5/10.

In three cases (5.26%), mild corneal edema was noted, with complete resolution under medical treatment.

Postoperative anterior uveitis was noted in seven patients (12.28%) who responded positively to medical treatment. In one of them, uveitis was present before IOL fixation; therefore we consider that our procedure reactivated it, rather than produced it.

Cystoid macular edema (CME) was identified in three cases (5.26%).

In one case, we had to reposition the IOL, due to high astigmatism (−6D) caused by IOL tilt, with good final outcome: BCVA 7/10.

Chronic glaucoma requiring long-term topical treatment was diagnosed in three patients in our series (5.26%), all within the trauma group.

We report no chronic corneal edema, no retinal detachment, and no suture break with subsequent IOL dislocation in the postoperative period in this series.

Uncorrected visual acuity improved in all cases within this series. BCVA of 5/10 or better was noted in 22 cases (38.59%). **Table 3** shows BCVA at the last control visit (3 months after surgery).

3.5 Discussion

Recovery of the visual function in an aphakic patient is challenging. Aphakic glasses are not an option, because of their high magnification and subsequent aniseikonia [4]. Contact lenses are difficult to handle, especially in older patients (medium age in our group was 64.22 years) who have never worn them before. Therefore, the only viable option in these cases is to place an IOL inside the eye. Since the capsular support is not adequate for IOL placement in the bag or in the sulcus, the available placement possibilities are anterior chamber, iris fixation (in its extreme or mid-periphery), or suture at the sclera.

Scleral fixation of an IOL is a safe option, and therefore it is the most used one in our practice. This preference is also explained by the fact that a vitreoretinal feels more comfortable working around pars plana and behind the iris plane, as compared to the AC.

The medium age of our patients (64.22 years) is higher as reported in the literature [4]. This might be partially explained by the high number of cases with previous complicated cataract surgeries (42.10%), since we are a referral center in the area. However, the medium age within the group with complicated cataract surgery is not significantly higher than within the trauma group: 65.20 years vs. 61.10 years, respectively. One observation is that five patients with posttraumatic IOL dislocation in the vitreous cavity were included in the trauma group, contributing to the increase of the medium age in this group.

As expected, men accounted for the majority of trauma cases: 24/30 (80%). In the group with complicated cataract surgery, male predominance, even if not so obvious, was still identified: 15/24 (62.50%).

3.5.1 Comments related to the IOL

In all cases we used the IOL model CZ70BD (Alcon, Fort Worth, Texas) (**Figure 1**). This is a rigid PMMA IOL. Foldable IOLs designed for sclera fixation were not available.

Since this IOL has only two eyelets, two-point fixation technique has been used in all cases. Therefore, it is more susceptible to IOL tilt which leads to higher-order aberrations that cannot be corrected with eyeglasses. In our series, in one single case we had to reposition a tilted IOL that determined high astigmatism (6D). Final outcome, after repositioning the IOL, was favorable, with BCVA 7/10.

Studies comparing the tilt concluded that it was significantly higher in SFIOL patients than in the ones with IOL in-the-bag [5].

Another IOL designed for being sutured at the sclera, Akreos AO 60 (Bausch & Lomb, Rochester, NY), has four haptics, each with its own eyelet for suture passage. The four-point fixation is theoretically associated with a lesser risk of tilt and dislocation, though there is no study comparing the differences in tilt between CZ70BD and Akreos AO 60 so far [6, 7]. Another major difference between the two implants is that Akreos AO 60 is hydrophilic and therefore susceptible to optic opacification by calcium salt deposition in case of air or gas filling of the eye [8]. Since the probability of future PPVs followed by internal tamponade in these complex cases is not negligible, Akreos AO 60 is not the optimal choice for these patients.

IOL dislocation following suture breakage is one serious complication, and it determines sudden visual drop. Since the last reported control visit in our patients is 3 months, the risk of this complication is still present, especially as most studies report it between 2 and 5 years after surgery [9]. The 10–0 polypropylene sutures that we used in all our patients are designated for sewing and ligation soft tissues in cardiovascular, neurological, and ophthalmic surgeries. Even if these sutures are firm and durable, there are reports indicating that they might not be a long-term solution to fixate an IOL [9]. Therefore, some surgeons recommend the use of 9–0 polypropylene sutures in these circumstances. Nevertheless, suture breakage was reported even with this type of sutures, especially in young adults and children [9]. An issue of concern related to the 9–0 polypropylene suture is related to the size of the knot. A bigger knot is associated with a higher risk of sclera atrophy, erosion, and resultant endophthalmitis [9]. This drawback is overcome by creating the sclera flaps covering the knots or by using an intrascleral Z suture instead of the knot [4].

When evaluating a surgical procedure in ophthalmology, there are two important interferingly elements to discuss: its impact on visual acuity and the complications related to it.

3.5.2 Visual acuity

In our series, BCVA of 5/10 or better was noted in 22 cases (38.59%). This is lower than reported by other authors [4, 10, 11], but the difference is that we did not exclude from our study the patients with associated lesions: RD, IOFB, and ruptured globe. In these circumstances, the final functional prognosis is influenced not only by IOL implantation technique but mainly by the consequences of other major ocular injuries.

The main advantage of surgery was that uncorrected visual acuity improved in every case in our series.

3.5.3 Complications

Since we used the infusion line of the PPV system, we were able to manage intraoperatively soft eye which may have had serious implications on functional recovery. Also, AC opening was performed cautiously, avoiding its sudden decompression which might have favored choroidal bleeding and detachment. The pars plana-placed infusion line allowed the maintenance of a relatively constant IOP throughout surgery.

We fashioned the sclera flaps before opening the AC, because the eye was more stable. Creating these flaps, even if laborious, is a very important step, aimed to increase the postoperative comfort of the patient and decrease the risk of endophthalmitis by burying the knots under them, which we did in all cases. Therefore, we report no case of postoperative endophthalmitis in this series.

Hemorrhage during surgery occurred in 20/57 cases (35.08%), and it was mild/moderate and self-limiting. It was produced during puncturing the sclera with the PC9 needle in all cases. This maneuver is performed "blindly" without actually seeing the tip of the needle but rather "feeling" it in its way through the sclera.

In the postoperative period, hemorrhage persisted in 10 cases (17.54%) but resolved spontaneously in 9 of them. In one case we had to reoperate the patient by PPV, 4 weeks after IOL suturing, since the hemorrhage had no tendency to clear. Final outcome was positive, with visual acuity of 5/10.

Postoperative astigmatism varied between −1.00D. cyl and -6D. cyl. The causes of astigmatism are corneal incision which is larger than in circumstances in which foldable IOLs are used, tight sutures, and IOL misalignment or tilt [3]. As previously mentioned, the high astigmatism due to IOL tilt forced us to reposition the IOL in only one situation that resolved positively, with final VA 7/10. Astigmatism could be significantly reduced by using foldable lenses for scleral fixation that can be inserted through smaller incisions.

Iris manipulation when fixating an IOL to the sclera is definitely more intense than when placing a foldable IOL in the bag; therefore an inherent complication is anterior uveitis, which we encountered in seven cases in our series (12.28%), a lower percentage than we found in the literature [3, 9]. Anterior uveitis responded promptly to medical therapy and resolved within 2–4 weeks after surgery.

CME was identified in three cases (5.26%) and prevented the increase of visual acuity. One possible explanation for it might be IOL instability inside the eye [2].

3.5.4 Advantages of scleral-fixated IOLs

One major advantage of scleral-fixated IOL, especially for a vitreoretinal surgeon, is that any future vitreoretinal surgery procedure can be performed with no risk of IOL dislocation, as may happen in anterior placed IOLs [12]. Moreover, these complicated cases in which secondary IOLs are indicated are at risk to develop posterior segment complications that require proper examination and even surgical treatment. Pupil dilatation and examination of the retina and vitreous are much easier in an eye with scleral-fixated IOL than in one with ACIOL or iris-fixated IOL [12]. Besides, PPV which is usually performed before suturing IOL at the sclera considerably decreases the risk of future posterior segment complications in these patients.

In all our cases, prior to suturing IOL at the sclera, PPV has been performed. This contributed to visual function improvement by eliminating all the debris, blood, and inflammatory cells from the vitreous cavity which are specific for the posttraumatic and complicated postcataract surgery settings [12].

Scleral-fixated IOL should be the preferred technique to correct aphakia also because it is more physiological than anterior segment IOL placement, which may be associated with the risk of corneal touch and loss of endothelium, anterior uveitis, and glaucoma in the long run [5]. Chronic glaucoma requiring long-term topical treatment was diagnosed in three patients in our series (5.26%), all in the trauma group, which allows us to speculate that posttraumatic injuries, rather than the surgical technique itself, were more likely to cause it.

Some surgeons advocate that in experienced hands, fixating an IOL to the sclera offers a visual prognosis which is good enough to favor this procedure as the standard of care for correcting aphakia in patients with insufficient capsular support [12]. With its limitations and lack of long-term follow-up, our study supports this idea. Larger sample and longer-term follow-up are necessary to establish the safety and complications associated with scleral-fixated IOLs. Also, there is room for innovating IOL designs and surgical techniques, like sutureless glueless scleral fixation IOL [13].

4. Conclusions

Ab interno scleral fixation of a rigid IOL was a safe and viable technique to correct aphakia in patients with inappropriate capsular support in this series.

During surgery, the most frequent complication was mild vitreous hemorrhage which was self-limiting and did not prevent the recovery of visual acuity.

The complications noted in the postoperative period were few and did not influence the overall visual prognosis.

The limitations of this study are the relatively small sample of patients and the short-term follow-up.

Studies on higher number of patients and with longer follow-up are mandatory in order to outline the status of scleral-fixated IOL as the standard of care for correcting aphakia in patients with insufficient capsular support.

Acknowledgements

Not applicable.
No funding.

Conflict of interest

The author declares no conflict of interest related to the publication of this paper.

Author details

Simona-Delia Nicoară
"Iuliu Hațieganu" University of Medicine and Pharmacy, Emergency County Hospital, Cluj-Napoca, Romania

*Address all correspondence to: simonanicoara1@gmail.com

IntechOpen

© 2019 The Author(s). Licensee IntechOpen. This chapter is distributed under the terms of the Creative Commons Attribution License (http://creativecommons.org/licenses/by/3.0), which permits unrestricted use, distribution, and reproduction in any medium, provided the original work is properly cited.

References

[1] Wagoner MD, Cox TA, Ariyasu RG, Jacobs DS, Karp CL, American Academy of Ophthalmology. Intraocular lens implantation in the absence of capsular support: A report by the American Academy of ophthalmology. Ophthalmology. 2003;**110**(4):840-859

[2] Brennan K. It's (Not) in the Bag: IOL Fixation. Review of Ophthalmology [Internet]. Available from: https://www.reviewofophthalmology.com/article/its-not-in-the-bag-iol-fixation

[3] Stem MS, Todorich B, Woodward MA, Hsu J, Wolfe JD. Scleral-fixated intraocular lenses: Past and present. Journal of VitreoRetinal Diseases. 2017;**1**(2):144-152. DOI: 10.1177/2474126417690650

[4] Reddy JML. Scleral fixation IOL: Outcome and complications. Journal of Evolution of Medical and Dental Sciences. 2016;**5**(20):991-993. DOI: 10.14260/jemds/2016/230

[5] Hayashi K, Hayashi H, Nakao F, Hayashi F. Intraocular lens tilt and decentration, anterior chamber depth, and refractive error after trans-scleral suture fixation surgery. Ophthalmology. 1999;**106**(5):878-882. DOI: 10.1016/S0161-6420(99)00504-7

[6] Fass ON, Herman WK. Four-point suture scleral fixation of a hydrophilic acrylic IOL in aphakic eyes with insufficient capsule support. Journal of Cataract and Refractive Surgery. 2010;**36**(6):991-996. DOI: 10.1016/j.jcrs.2009.12.043

[7] Fass ON, Herman WK. Sutured intraocular lens placement in aphakic post-vitrectomy eyes via small-incision surgery. Journal of Cataract and Refractive Surgery. 2009;**35**(9):1492-1497. DOI: 10.1016/j.jcrs.2009.04.034

[8] Cao D, Zhang H, Yang C, Zhang L. Akreos adapt AO intraocular lens opacification after vitrectomy in a diabetic patient: A case report and review of the literature. BMC Ophthalmology. 2016;**16**:82. DOI: 10.1186/s12886-016-0268-3

[9] Wasiluk E, Krasnicki P, Dmuchowska DA, Proniewska-Skretek E, Mariak Z. The implantation of the scleral-fixated posterior chamber intraocular lens with 9/0 polypropylene sutures–long-term visual outcomes and complications. Advances in Medical Sciences. 2019;**64**(1):100-103

[10] Lee VY, Yuen HK, Kwok AK. Comparison of outcomes of primary and secondary implantation of sclera fixated posterior chamber intraocular lens. The British Journal of Ophthalmology. 2003;**87**(12):1459-1462. DOI: 10.1136/bjo.87.12.1459

[11] Ghanem VC, Ghanem EA, Ghanem RC. Monoscleral fixation IOL after extra capsular extraction of subluxated lenses in patients with Marfan syndrome. Arquivos Brasileiros de Oftalmologia. 2004;**64**:763-767. DOI: org/10.1590/S0004-27492004000500013

[12] Saxena D, Patel C. Visual outcome in scleral fixated intraocular lenses. Journal of Evolution of Medical and Dental Sciences. 2016;**5**(55):3716-3717. DOI: 10.14260/jemds/2016/852

[13] Cheung CS, VanderVeen DK. Intraocular lens techniques in pediatric eyes with insufficient capsular support: Complications and outcomes. Seminars in Ophthalmology. 2019;**34**(4):293-302

CPSIA information can be obtained
at www.ICGtesting.com
Printed in the USA
LVHW050750040423
743361LV00003B/366

9 781838 804848